Chinese Medicine & Healthcare
Centre
24 Bernard Street, Leith
Edinburgh EH6 6PP
Tel. 0131 554 7888

GUIDE TO TRADITIONAL CHINESE MEDICINE

GUIDE TO TRADITIONAL CHINESE MEDICINE

Raymond R Bullock

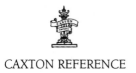

CAXTON REFERENCE

© 2001 Caxton Editions

This edition published 2001 by Caxton Publishing Group Ltd,
20 Bloomsbury Street, London, WC1B 3JH.

Design and compilation by The Partnership Publishing Solutions Ltd,
Glasgow, G77 5UN

Printed and bound in India

DISCLAIMER

This book is meant to be an introduction to
Traditional Chinese Medicine – it's only purpose is to
induce the interested reader to seek out a qualified
practitioner, and find out more. It is the author's
belief that TCM can neither be taught, nor passed on
through the written word – this book does not
attempt to do either.

It is important to note that TCM practitioners do
not claim TCM to be a substitute for orthodox
medical treatment, but do suggest that it can be used
to complement all treatments, whether they are
conventional or alternative therapies. Therefore, it is
recommended that the reader discuss his or her
condition with their GP, and attain their guidance,
before attempting other methods.

Many of the theories and concepts in this book,
especially for related therapies, are the result of
research and not necessarily the opinions of the
author or publishers.

ABOUT THE AUTHOR

Raymond R Bullock is a poet and writer from the
Wirral, currently teaching T'ai Ji Quan, martial arts,
and Oriental poetry and philosophy. He also promotes
group studies in stress reduction through
contemplative writing and T'ai Chi exercises.

After studying at John Moores University in
Liverpool he received a degree in Philosophy and
Imaginative Writing and a Master's degree in Writing.

His interest in Chinese philosophy and related arts
ranges over a thirty-year period, and centres on the
study of the I Ching and its use as an instrument in
self-development.

Writing interests at the present time include, a
collection of Haiku poems and Writing as Therapy.
His account of the I Ching is published by Caxton
Editions in the current series.

GRATITUDE LIST

My thanks firstly to Gill Hayes and Pat Power for use of their centre for photographs. The Centre For Holistic Therapies, the Blackwell Building in Brook Street, Neston on the Wirral (CH649XJ), can be contacted via phone on 0151336 6222 or at:

cht@hol-therapy.com and www.hol-therapy.com

Further thanks to Annette C Smith for standing in as model for the pictures. To Stephen and Vicki Hon for the photo and computer graphics. My thanks to authors and publishers, mentioned in the bibliography and throughout the book, without whom my understanding of TCM and other therapies would be much narrower.

Thanks also to Professor Yee of the Water's Edge Holistic Centre, for various and many occasions of support and guidance. Most especially for the translation of the T'ai Chi Classic, Chi Gung closing exercise, and for much of my interest in TCM and its connection with the I Ching.

Thanks last but not least, to Kam Lau my T'ai Chi instructor, and to Grandmaster Chen Xiaowang, for my continued interest and understanding of Tai Chi.

DEDICATION

I dedicate this book to Jane, Carol, Michelle and Allan for their love and unconditional support; my life is brighter for their presence. Also to Becky, Ashleigh, Adam, Danny, Brandon and all further grandchildren to appear after this book is published, for the same.

Contents

Introduction

Chinese Traditional Medicine is an ancient art of healing. Its roots can be traced back into antiquity. So far in fact that much of its origins are undocumented. We therefore depend on supposition and mythology to explain the genesis of its primary aspects, acupuncture, massage and herbalism. Because these began many hundreds of years before the written word, we can only assume that somewhere in the mythology are the connections we are looking for to explain how such a diverse medicine came about.

The origins of any Herbalism are obviously linked to diet; in the search for food man noticed that one thing would cause excess heat in the stomach, while another removed it. This information was shared, until it became common knowledge.

As societies formed, the position of healer or Shaman became one of importance, and they depended on him/her to provide cures for all levels of disease. The Shaman provided herbs for use in two main ways: internally for purification and the removal of toxins, and externally for the treatment of wounds etc.

In the ancient Chinese book 'Shen Nong's herbal classic', more than fifty per cent of the 365 medicines listed, stressed dietary as well as medicinal significance.

There is a legend that Shen Nong tested hundreds of plants and herbs every day and was poisoned many times, but his medical knowledge was so great that he was always able to heal himself. By medical knowledge we mean, he understood the human condition and its changes so well, that he was able to restore balance with the use of his potions.

Centuries later in the T'ang dynasty Meng Shen wrote 'The Dietetic Materia Medica' in which most of the material was made up of the daily food requirements. Fruit and vegetables, both wild and cultivated, cereals, game and poultry, seafood – including seaweed shrimp and shellfish, herbs and more were given as examples of 'materia medica' and therefore as primary sources of health and balance.

Acupuncture's origins, it is claimed, are simpler, because of the links to pain.

After standing on a sharp stone or thorn a man might find that there was a lack of feeling in some other area of the body. By pressing a thorn into that part of the foot on other occasions the result would be repeated, and if he pressed another part of the foot a similar result occurred in some further part of the body.

The first needles used by Shamans were reputedly made of stone, then animal bones and finally as society progressed, of metal.

Primarily used as an anaesthetic, the healer could reset a dislocated shoulder for instance, by placing a needle in the area of the knee. He/she could then use manipulation (massage) on the affected area, and finally apply an herbal treatment to affect a cure.

Twisting or even breaking the ankle required a needle to be placed between the thumb and index finger, followed again by manipulation and herbal medication.

A further example would be in the case of an unsettled stomach, where the acupuncture point would be three fingers down on the wrist.

Manipulation, or massage, also has simple and obvious beginnings; touch being the most basic way in which animals and man receive comfort.

As with Reiki, Tui Na is a safe form of therapy. If in practise the pressure is not at the correct point, then no damage results. There will of course be no healing either, because the chi/blood flow will not have been affected.

Stress is one of the major causes of serious illness and Tui Na is extremely effective in this area. Stress manifests in many ways and relaxation is one way of relieving it, but Tui Na can go further than this by manipulating the flow of chi, thereby treating the problem at the subtle energy level.

Sports and health centres are an expanding industry. Many millions of people each week are involved in fitness techniques of one form or another. The physical stresses that come with this kind of activity often end up with muscle and joint injuries and sprains. Tui Na is particularly useful here because it not only treats the damaged area, but also helps to increase vitality and stimulate the immune system through its holistic viewpoint.

In each of these aspects of TCM the primary thing is to find the yang condition or the yin condition, and push the whole organism in the direction of balance. This is the holistic viewpoint.

The meridian system covers the whole of the body and is cyclic; it has no beginning and no end. It represents the pathways in which the chi, or life force, circulates freely throughout the body. (Chi is like the motor force that drives the blood.) When there is a blockage of chi, the balance is lost and will result in what we describe as disease, but what Chinese medicine more simply describes as an excess or deficiency of yin or yang. The blockage might have a psychological, chemical or biological cause but the solution begins with the restoration of chi circulation.

This meridian system is a part of what Dr. Yee calls the self-organizing body-system (as explained in the forward), through which the human organism constantly seeks to realign the balancing forces of yin and yang.

The basic philosophy here is that the individual is an ecological unit, reflecting the ecosystem in which he or she lives. The maintenance of health in both is achieved through the restoration of balance before the damage is too great: prevention is always better than cure. Living a balanced life, in preference to one of excess or constant deprivation, is the holistic solution.

A good physician cures the patient, a great physician shows him how to prevent disease.

The balanced life, according to TCM, is the natural (or centred) one. The excessive lifestyle of the twentieth century, and its resultant conditions, is a demonstration of the TCM paradigm described above.

The principal teaching of ancient Chinese philosophy, as illustrated in the I Ching, is self-development. Self-development is overall balance and therefore includes physical health. The teaching of the sage-kings was based on practical holistic principles:

Know the enemy and know the self...

Disease could be prevented if one knew and understood the internal and external forces, and how these could be manipulated for optimum health. This is what Dr. Yee terms – spontaneous healing behaviour.

When the yin/yang condition is so far out of balance that the self-organizing body-system cannot easily return it to its natural equilibrium, either premature death or severe debility occurs. This can then only be altered through conscious knowledge of the condition. This book describes ways in which ancient and modern Chinese doctors used knowledge of their environment: of how they fitted in to it, and the ways in which balance could be restored.

Of equal importance to the sage-kings was that self-development be shared with others so that they too could benefit. The philosophy here was also practical – if individuals were responsible for their own well-being they would not become dependent, and therefore burdens, upon society. Society would also not become a draining force upon the environment.

The purpose of this book is to demonstrate that each of us can learn simple techniques to aid in living a fuller and more natural lifestyle. Also that in accepting this responsibility and applying some of the techniques, we will have made a beginning in the journey of self-development.

Foreword
by Zude Yee

To the Chinese, China is Zhong Gui. Zhong Gui means Central Kingdom.

In the study of Chinese culture, we should understand why the Chinese call their country Zhong Gui.

Zhong portrays the fundamental worldview of the Chinese. The primary meaning of Zhong is balance, and can be perceived in the following ways:

Ancient Chinese culture recognised the four cardinal points of east, west, south and north and that China was at the centre.
It was therefore, in perfect balance.

It was also a fundamental part of this philosophy that heaven was above and earth below with man in the middle. Heaven was round (a circle) and earth square with man again at the centre.

Chinese philosophy expresses a neutral policy toward everything: relationship should be balanced. In daily life, one should be neither too full nor too hungry; dressed not too warm or too cold, and ones reactions ought to be neither hurried or slow.

Walking is called Zhong Bu meaning a balanced step. The Taoists stress Zhong Kon, which translates as 'empty in the middle'. Confucius' paradigm was Zhong Yuong or essential balance.

Health is Balance, keeping fit is to keep balance; illness is unbalanced; treatment is restoring balance.

Tai chi is centred balance; Chi gung is Guan Zhong meaning watching the centre or Sou Zhong, which is keeping centred.

What we suggest to the reader is to keep this word, Zhong in your memory because it is important for the study of anything Chinese. The understanding of TCM will be made much easier by knowing and appreciating its implications.

Therefore the first and simplest definition of TCM is: Balancing medicine or more specifically Energy Balancing Medicine.

Dynamic Balancing

The ancient Chinese understood that balance was an ideal situation. They knew that for the body-physical, reality was a constantly shifting situation. It was an adjustment, from balance to unbalance and back again. They understood that:

In the real world, nothing is absolute – nothing holds perfect balance.

The I Ching says,

Observe stillness in movement, movement in stillness.

This of course, is the essence of tai chi, whose source is to found in the philosophy of the I Ching. Things are always in a state of flux, forever moving, however slowly, however imperceptibly, from one extreme to the other. In ancient Chinese thought, the seeds of balance are to be found when things are at their most unstable, and vice versa.

This means that when a condition or movement is at the extreme of yang, it becomes yin; when the condition has reached extreme yin it becomes yang. In TCM it might require help to bring this about.

In the history of human beings medicine is a recent introduction, but there can have been very few cultures where it does not have a major influence.

Being dependent upon its resources we might wonder how they survived before medicine. The answer is simple to Taoist thinking: whether because God created life, or if we prefer, as a result of evolution, mankind has a fixed self-healing system. This self-healing system includes self-organization and spontaneous healing behaviour. These two aspects are used in different ways to control the unbalancing process.

Let's simply draw a line: the dynamic balance has a range, say, between point A and point B. Where the balance shifts between A and B, we call this 'the dynamic range'. In this situation the human body has a function, which is constantly returning the body toward a state of equilibrium, or health. Activating this function is a system, which we call self-organization.

Self-organization is the body-system, which activates control of the dynamic balancing of the human organism. This means that our self-organization is always in action and we need not worry about our balance – as long as the balance does not shift out of the line we have drawn between A and B.

Compensation is what we call the bridge or process, which connects balancing with unbalancing.

Our second aspect, Spontaneous Self-healing Behaviour, means to deal with that unbalancing, which is beyond the range of the dynamic process A and B.

In this stage people feel discomfort as they start to suffer. The body's reaction or impulse is to seek some way to halt the suffering, outside of the normal compensatory process.

This behaviour we call spontaneous healing behaviour, which includes most of Traditional Chinese Medicine's approaches. It is spontaneous in that its appearance is instinctive, being imperative for survival. Behaviour implies action, but while the origins of the behaviour are unconscious, i.e. spontaneous, intelligence and consciousness make it possible to build on this foundation and use nature and natural forces to achieve re-balance.

For example, if we examine spontaneous healing-behaviour as the origin of Tuina, acupuncture and Herbal medicine, we might come up with examples like the following.

Tuina

TCM massage is called Tuina. Tuina indicates two main manipulations of Chinese massage:

Tui- is pushing the muscle. As we know, touching by animals or human beings is a fundamental way of relieving pain. Without thinking your hands will press on the area and start to rub. This means that there is no argument that massage originated from spontaneous healing behaviour.

-Na is another essential Chinese massage manipulation: the act of grasping muscle. Such powerful manipulation our ancestors used to control the pain in the areas rich in muscle. Here again is evidence that massaging originated from spontaneous healing behaviour.

TCM still uses its herbs in their rough, crude, natural shape. It has become fashionable in the West for some people to take the herbs in this old style without preparation: the dried plant parts: root, branch, leafs, and flowers cooked with water and drunk the same as tea. In modern herbal industries, the refined products may have some speciality, but the old style has been proved for thousands of years.

Herbs are a funny tasting food: sour, bitter, salt or pungent. They are unlike the normal food focus, which is mainly on sweet-tastes. We have reason to believe that the herbal healing started from diet management.

Suppose there was one ancestor who found that if he ate sour food, the stomach heat disappeared: we can say this is spontaneous – meaning without conscious or special motivation – he becomes consciously aware now that the sour tasting food make the heat go from the stomach, and he may repeat the experiment over and over again. This is, of course, the way of science.

On the other hand he might also have found that if he took sweet food it could make his stomach heat much worse, and so he learnt to avoid this type of food. It was in this way that he found how to manage his trouble.

After he made sure his experience was true, he shared this knowledge with his relatives and friends. Knowledge piece by piece was collected in this way, over thousands of years. The result is today's Chinese herbal medicine.

Spontaneous healing is a basic survival skill of animal behaviour. Massage is the first spontaneous healing response, plants and diet the second. A parent's touch to comfort and heal comes naturally to us. The body sends out craving impulses for certain foods at certain times.

We will argue now that acupuncture is also an act of spontaneous healing.

Students in Totnes, Exeter, Manchester, Perth and New Brighton (Liverpool), who know how to use 'Fractal Acupuncture' already believe so. They have all experienced a 'magic' training, in a few minutes. They have quickly become Fractal Acupuncturists who can administer the fractal needle to cope with their suffering.

The simple system of treatment has been used for asthma, Parkinson's Disease, psoriasis, prostrate conditions, period pains and other difficult illnesses. Asthma sufferers stop using the inhaler, during an attack. They simply use the Fractal needle method to puncture a particular point, and in no more than two minutes, the breath returns back to normal.

When I was young, in the Gobi Desert, we were barefoot, working in the field. The earth's ruggedness always made the feet swollen, itchy, and burning. Then my grandfather showed us how to use a sharp needle from a plant, to puncture the foot and relieve the pain. That was my first acupuncture experience: simple, easy, and practical.

Human behaviour is always focused on expanding on our environment. We obsess with complicating and enlarging things. We can compare this with the first acupuncture book, which was initially a very small book. Some 2000 years later, influenced by so-called reductionist science, an acupuncture manual is a huge, complicated affair. Acupuncture has changed its face, but it doesn't have to be this way, as the one needle Fractal Acupuncture approach proves beyond doubt.

Humans make the theory – nature makes the garden.

TCM – as simple as common sense

The human body is a complex system.

The Yellow Emperor's summary was compiled over 2000 years ago.

At that time there was no physiology or biology but people were still born, grew up and died. Before they died they would of course, have had a lot of suffering. For life to be easy, with less suffering, the ancient sages found ways to deal with all kind of illness.

The original ideas about health are encompassed in just four words in Chinese:

Cei - means eating well: meaning a balanced diet. Neither too hungry, nor too full.

He -means to drink without being too thirsty, or drinking too much.

La- is defined as, ones stool should be neither painfully dry nor diarrhoea. Urinate, not too much or too little, too dark or too light.

Sui- means to sleep well. Not for too long or suffering from insomnia. When arising, being full of energy.

These four principles are still today, the Chinese farmers health standards. Being born in the countryside on a farm, I know them well. We lived in the simplest nature, without big dreams. What life gave was what we received. Without great expectations there were no major disappointments and therefore no emotional problems.

Thus if those four basic conditions are good, the person can be considered healthy.

Now we will extend our conceptualisation of health by another word: Tong meaning pain.

A healthy body should be comfortable and without pain. If there is pain, this indicates something is wrong. But the Chinese explain that pain is simple and reasonable to understand. Pain is caused by stagnation. The stagnation may involve chi or blood.

Chi is such a special concept in Chinese philosophy that we will have to describe it in more detail later. Here we will give only a general definition, which is that it is the vital energy.

In Chinese, chi also means air. Therefore, if the pain involves chi, the patients should feel the pain of swelling. Also chi moves easily, so that chi stagnation, which is causing the pain, may move from one place to another, along with the pain.

Blood, in Chinese medicine, is also different to the common meaning. Here we must firstly take the concept of blood as the general one. That is - real blood.

If the blood stagnates, Chinese medicine calls it Dead Blood. This dead blood cannot move, so when the pain is caused by blood stagnation, the pain is always fixed at its location, and the pain sounds like the needle pinking.

All the TCM principles can be understood in this

common sense basis.

Common sense never changes, and so TCM has lasted thousands of years. Its principles still work today, and we may confidently surmise they will continue to work for another thousands of years.

Since, as we have seen, TCM comes from spontaneous healing behaviour, and can be understood from a common sense base, we can perceive that TCM is easy and simple to learn.

If you learn from the systems aspects, rather than the current college study methods, in my experience one years training part time, plus your own extensive hard work, is enough to let you enter and master TCM's main approaches.

CHAPTER I
Perspectives

East and West (Yin and Yang)

The primary difficulties in the assimilation of cross-cultural knowledge lie in the perspectives of those cultures. A society functions in the way that it views reality and this viewpoint is shaped by its belief system. The problem of accepting new ideas depends on how well they fit in with the present perspective, and so in the first chapter of this book we ought to aim at recognising and removing these barriers.

The Chinese perspective is evident in the way that the TCM practitioner deals with his patient. He diagnoses the whole person: the personal and family history, environment, and diet and present behaviour patterns. He will observe skin-tone and posture; listen to voice and breath and even ask for a sample of handwriting. All of this he will do in order to diagnose disorders before they become major problems.

These observations and many more he will view as exterior expressions of internal conditions.

The Western perspective involves treating the problem as it becomes manifest.

Chinese medicine is pretty much the same in the third millennium as it was four thousand years ago. It is what its name implies – a Traditional medicine. In Chinese medicine the patient is shown how to heal himself, in Western medicine the patient is dependent on the doctor.

Western medical science on the other hand, is forever expanding. It is dynamic and creative. Science continues to expand at a phenomenal rate, encompassing areas bordering on the miraculous.

Western medicine, because of this creativity, as well as its vast store of knowledge can do no less than demand a dependency from its patients; this is its yang nature. Chinese medicine, with its Traditionalism is yin and therefore its patients are required to take responsibility for their own well-being.

Up until the middle ages Western Europeans viewed their reality in a similar way to the Chinese: they had a direct connection to the world and the universe through Nature and God. Nature governed what could be perceived via the senses and God governed the unseen, the numinous. The split from this way of thinking came from the great philosophers, primarily Aristotle and Descartes.

Matter was permanent and the laws of Nature were fixed, therefore man could know and control matter if he knew the laws. To Renee Descartes the world and the universe was a machine, meaning that man as a part of this reality was also a mechanical instrument. A machine has many different parts. Yes, they are all connected to the whole thing – the machine – but each can be replaced or dealt with separately.

This systematic reductive reasoning eventually led to the idea that mechanistic problems could be predicted, that all machines suffered from the same foreseeable maladies and could all be treated in the same manner.

The only analysis necessary was of the disease itself; all patients were pretty much the same.

This provided the need for a new industry – mass production of remedies was the new way. It was the beginning of the cause and effect mind set of modern medicine. If the cause of the problem were isolated it could be cut out or a simple solution found. There was no need for any further analysis.

The major problem in avoiding this particular philosophy is that the solutions work. Insulin, a modern miracle cure, works to increase the insulin not provided by the pancreas in some sufferers. Diabetes is a killer, yet sufferers no longer die. Ergo the science of cause and effect is validated. No more analysis is necessary. The natural strength and weaknesses of the individual are not taken into account.

A Chinese doctor, in dealing with Western medicine as an entity, would say it was too yang and prescribe a little yin. The yin is to accept a synthesis of Eastern medicine, just as Chinese medicine has accepted a synthesis of Western medicine.

The division of mind and body, again from Descartes, has become something other than what the great philosopher had in mind. Man has assumed power over nature, it seems, but in order to believe this he must deny the holistic nature of his whole being. To separate the one from the other and create a dualist reality is not to deny either one. Descartes reality is the reality of the Western world, and this reality is about power.

Conversely, to depend on a myriad of outside forces i.e. powerful spirits, is equally disempowering. When myth creates gods on which to depend, as well as to blame, then a world has been created in which no action can be taken to further individuals or peoples in their growth.

Scientific medicine and traditional Chinese medicine is about self-development, one from one point of view and one from another. Science is yang, TCM is yin: for us in the West a synthesis of both would be balance.

Yin and Yang

Yin and yang are complementary opposite forces, through whose interaction life is created. They are the energies of heaven and earth.

The oldest Chinese ideograms for yin and yang both depict the side of a mountain. Yang includes an image of the sun and its rays and yin includes a cloud. When the side of a mountain has more sunlight it is yang, but as the cloud moves across the sky creating shadow, it becomes yin. When our energies are vibrant we are yang, if tranquil, we are yin. Remember that as the energy changes so does our yin or yang-ness.

Throughout the body the yang meridians channel the energy of heaven downward, and the energy of earth, through yin meridians, upward.

In simple terms sunlight, the creative yang energy, mixes with the earth, the receptive yin energy and plants and animals are born. Neither yin nor yang exists without the other, and so everything in the universe is made of varying degrees of each. They constantly interact and depend, one upon the other. Between them they create the qualities of things.

The famous yin/yang symbol, which looks like two fish, one dark, one light, forever following each other is probably the best illustration of how this particular concept works. Within each side is the seed of the other, like day and night, summer and winter. At the point of most light, the summer solstice, winter has begun its imperceptible march across the land. The winter solstice is the birth of the new light and so on.

The symbol represents the self-organizing body system, described by Dr. Yee in the Foreword. In such a system change and adaptation are of primary importance for survival.

The ancients viewed change via the four seasons, and from this came the philosophy of the five elements, or five stages, of change.

Keeping in mind the simple image of the yin/yang symbol, we can observe how the seasons change from one stage into the next: Yin is both autumn and winter and yang is spring and summer.

Spring is described as young yang, when the light energy awakens new life. Summer the energy becomes full. As in the fish symbol, the seeds of yin then become manifest, developing into autumn. After which yin becomes full in winter. This represents a dynamic cyclic movement.

Yang represents an expansive movement, energy bursting outward - from seed to fullness of growth. Yin is the opposing contraction of energies like the seed that waits beneath the soil.

The five elements (WU HSING), or stages of change are represented thus:

- Spring is **wood**
- Summer is **fire**
- Autumn is **metal**
- Winter is **water**.

Wood personifies young energies as the seed that breaks through the soil and grows to fullness.

Fire because the world is close to the sun, the source of heat and light.

Metal representing that, which is precious and condensed within the earth at this time.

Water symbolizes the energies or spirit of life sinking into the depths of the earth.

At the centre of this dynamic movement is the earth, which represents the fifth element.

The five elements each have a representative organ but we will discuss this later. For the moment we can demonstrate the five element (or five phase) theory thus:

FIRE

WOOD **EARTH** **METAL**

WATER

This is known as the Yellow River Map.

Yin and Yang and TCM analysis

In terms of TCM analysis, facial lines denote yin or yang life styles. Excessive amounts of sugars, liquid and fats create horizontal lines, while too much meat and salt cause vertical or yang lines.

Again, too much liquid is usually the cause of a nose, which is soft and swollen. This yin condition is an indication of an enlarged heart. An excess of milk products such as cheese and butter is indicated when the nose is swollen but hard. The result of this kind of diet is heart failure because of the inflexibility of the heart.

A demonstration of the dynamic natures of yin and yang in biological terms is as follows:

The primary systems of the human organism are the circulatory, the digestive and the nervous systems. When we are at the embryonic stage, yin in the form of the nervous system is on the outside, while yang formed by the digestive system is inside.

As the embryo develops these systems begin to change polarity. The outside yin attracts yang and hardens, while the inside yang attracts yin and softens. This outside yang develops into the back and spine while the yin of the inside becomes the internal organs.

Yin and Yang and Balance

Yin and yang are the complementary opposites whose interaction creates life. All things in the world and the universe have yin and yang characteristics. Our bodies have yin and yang features, for instance our internal organs. What the Chinese call Zhang organs are yin, while the Fu organs are yang (See Chapter 4 Zhang/Fu Organs). When these are balanced in their energies, we are healthy and when there is an excess or insufficiency we have ill-health.

The essential then is to understand how to return the body to yin/yang balance. As in Reiki (see my book Undertsanding Reiki - Physician heal thyself') there is an interchange between healer and recipient.

Chi (life-force) is perceived as an intelligent energy, which reaches the patient via the healer, who considers him/herself as a channel only. The communication between healer and patient, therefore, is both active and subtle. As we have stated, the significant interaction is on the energy level, but it is also important in TCM that the patient gives the therapist as much feedback as possible. This not only directs the therapist to the areas requiring treatment, but also indicates how much pressure to use.

Again, as with Reiki, the one who is the channel benefits as the subtle energies also enhance his/her own yin/yang balance.

CHAPTER 3
Vital Substances

In Chinese medicine the body has five vital substances: these are chi, blood, jing, shen, and the body fluids. Of these five chi (energy), shen (spirit) and jing (essence) are called the three treasures. The three treasures form the basis of the energy transformations of the body. They are interdependent and interactive.

Jing

Jing or essence is the most refined substance of our physical being. It regulates all physical growth, reproduction and development. We inherit original jing from our parents and it is the basis of our constitutional energy. (It should be noted that in TCM there is an important difference between a person's condition and constitution. The constitution is formed at conception, and is unalterable. Qualities and characteristics acquired after birth, such as skin tone can be altered by diet or life style. This is called the condition.)

The amount of jing received prior to birth is irreplaceable and so TCM practitioners recommend conserving what we have.

The jing is stored in the kidneys and is lost through too many pregnancies in women, and excessive sex (ejaculation) in men. Sperm is the bodily equivalent of jing and so ought to be preserved.

Shen

Shen is translated as spirit or spirits. The 'Yellow Emperor's Classic of Internal Medicine' proclaims the heart as the emotional and spiritual centre. The heart is 'The Ruler' or 'The Emperor' of the body, and this refers to the shen, which resides there. All of the organs have a spirit or shen , which is also translated as mind and consciousness.

As the ruling spirit, the shen of the heart works with the shen of the other organs, to strengthen the spiritual attributes: with the shen of the kidneys to understand the deeper meaning of life and for spiritual strength; with the shen of the liver for prophecy and strategic skills; with the shen of the lungs to balance the rhythms of the body and the breath; with the shen of the spleen to generate discernment.

Chi and blood

The organ governing the chi is the lung and the circulation of chi through the body coincides with the rhythm of the breath. Once we understand this, it becomes obvious why a Chinese doctor will recommend t'ai chi or chi gung to his patients. In either of these exercises the mind controls the breath, and therefore the circulation of chi, throughout the movements.

Blood is produced, in the heart and bone marrow, from the chi of our diet and breath. This blood/chi is carried through the veins to supply organs and tissues with vital energy and lubrication.

Blood is stored in the liver, where the quality and quantity are guarded if the liver is healthy. The opposite aspect of the liver function with regard to blood is that it promotes the free circulation of both blood and chi.

The systems of chi and blood are of primary importance. The chi, as we know, is the life force and the instigator of life. It is both a protector and a cultivator of growth. These are its male and female aspects.

Also the chi is the 'director of the blood' while the blood is the 'mother/nurturer' of chi. This describes how the chi and blood relate to each other. Chi is yang in relation to blood, and blood is yin in relation to chi. (Remember that Yin and Yang are relative concepts.)

Where there is an imbalance, a blockage occurs: the chi cannot drive the blood and blood cannot generate chi and so they stagnate in the channels. This causes disease and damage to the tissues and bones.

The chi flows through channels called meridians, energising the internal organs, mind and spirit. The balance or imbalance of yin and yang, meaning health or ill-health, manifests physically, mentally and emotionally, as well as spiritually.

Body fluids

The liquids that moisten the tissues, muscles, joints and organs of the body, as well as skin and hair are called jin and ye. Tears and sweat are jin, the rest are ye.

The kidneys control the balance of liquids: they assess quantity and quality throughout the body and are responsible for the prevention of excess or deficiency, whether through sweating, urination or tears.

CHAPTER 4
The Zang-fu and Extraordinary Organs

Immediately that we mention organs we receive a
pictorial image and something of their function, from
our memory banks. This is because, in the West, the
sciences of physiology and anatomy give us the only
view we know of our internal substance.

Knowing the function of these materials we can
restore them to normal condition when they go
wrong. 'When they go wrong', might require surgery,
drugs or even complete replacement, to restore
normal function. These and other solutions result
from viable scientific study, and a thorough
knowledge of physiology and anatomy.

In Chinese medicine, however, less emphasis is
placed on the individual function of the organs. The
emphasis is more on how and where each fits in to
the bodily energy process as a whole.

This holistic viewpoint pictures the body as a
dynamic process rather than a mechanical instrument.
From this perspective, the organs are seen as a part of

this process, rather than as separate structures functioning mechanically.

This is not to say that one of these attitudes is wrong and the other right, only that they are both extreme viewpoints. This being so, the viability of each cannot be determined from the opposite perspective.

We have suggested that Western medicine functions in a yang manner, while medicine of the East is more yin. In the philosophy of yin/yang, when one or the other gets too full, it begins to change to its opposite. It might seem this way with both forms of medicine, for each has begun to take on a little of the other. The main purpose of this primer is to give the beginner a general insight into the Eastern perspective.

This being so we can attempt to create a simple illustration of the yang fu organs and their function in TCM.

Zang Organs are **yin** and solid so they store but do not transmit. They are:

- **lungs**
- **heart**
- **spleen**
- **kidneys**
- **liver**
- Also the **pericardium** or Heart Protector, (a membranous sac enclosing the heart) which

TCM regards as part of the heart and not a separate organ.

Fu Organs are **yang** and hollow so they transform but cannot retain. They are:

- **small intestine**
- **large intestine**
- **stomach**
- **gall bladder**
- **bladder**
- Also the **sanjiao** or Triple Warmer, for which there is no Western anatomical equivalent. Again this is not a true organ but rather describes the passageway, through the abdomen, for fluids and chi.

There are also a series of less important organs known as **Extraordinary Fu**. These are:

- **brain**
- **marrow**
- **uterus**
- **bone**
- **blood vessels**
- And again the **gall bladder**, which is also Fu.

The five organ networks

Each network consists of its own set of functions and is named after its Zang or yin organ. Zang and Fu organs are paired together in each system, which contain both physiological and psychological aspects. Finally each organ has its own channel. This of course covers only ten of the twelve channels, the other two are named after the pericardium, (which the Chinese consider to be the active mechanism of the heart and not an organ in its own right) and the sanjiao or triple-warmer. The sanjiao is represented by the three bodily cavities of the chest, abdomen and pelvic area.

The paired organ networks are as follows:
- Liver and gallbladder
- Heart and small intestine
- Kidney and bladder
- Lung and large intestine
- Spleen and stomach

As we have stated the yin organs are solid and store chi, whereas the yang organs are hollow and transmit chi. Yin organs exhibit stability and constancy while the yang organs are dynamic and therefore less stable. Yin organs regulate the metabolism; temperature, pressure and distribution while the yang organs take care of digestion and elimination.

As well as maintaining the above essential

mechanisms, each network exhibits its own intellectual, emotional and behavioural character. Each character is represented in the five element (five phase) system.

Chinese philosophy is based on the principal that the energies governing change in the macrocosm also govern the microcosm: forces that empower the planets empower the human organism in the same way. The yearly cycle, as represented by the Yellow River Map, can also depict the human life cycle. Each phase of life has its own character and energy.

We can view this in the following way:

FIRE

heart/small intestine

WOOD　　　　**EARTH**　　　　**METAL**

liver/gall bladder　*sleen/stomach*　*lung/large intestine*

WATER

kidney/bladder

In the above sequence, the Water/Kidney element is at the base, which depicts the kidneys as the root of the bodily chi, and therefore of all of the organs. It represents the wellspring of human vitality and creativity.

The spleen holds central place, just as the earth does, both being the constant provider around which the others congregate for life and sustenance.

At the top is the heart as Emperor. It represents clarity and wisdom, which it shares unconditionally with its subjects. The expansive personality of the heart also depicts the nature of fire and summer. The life of the world depends on the energy of the sun for all areas of development and growth.

The liver collects and distributes blood and therefore chi, while the lung collects and distributes the chi. Both are mediators. The liver is like a general while the lung is a minister. Liver is spring and wood, bursting from the restraining soil and blackness of winter, following the line of least resistance. Lung is metal and autumn, taking only that which is vital into the earth.

We will now take a brief look at the various functions and processes of the Zang and Fu organs, including their distinct characters. Hopefully this will help the reader to view the body as a dynamic process.

Before we do so we will alter the River Map to demonstrate the Sheng and Ke cycles.

Sheng is the name for the cycle of promotion in which we follow the outside arrows. Ke is the cycle of control, following the inside arrows.

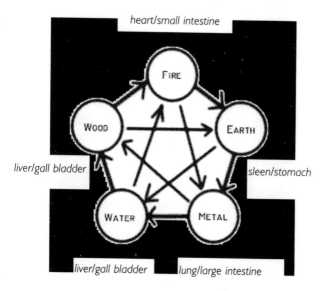

The heart network

The heart rules the Central Palace also known as the heart chakra. It is the spiritual and emotional centre from which our sense of well-being emanates. It drives the blood and stores the spirits. Shen in Chinese means spirit or spirits. Each of the organs has its own spirit but the heart has the controlling spirit.

In the ancient texts the Shen were simply the representatives of heaven, willing to influence the lives of men when asked. It was necessary to practise stillness, or meditation, in order to create an openness, through which they might enter.

Alternatively, the Shen can represent the multitude of spiritual, moral and psychological faculties. When the heart is healthy, its energies balanced and without stress, these higher faculties are also healthy and able to direct our lives. The true compassion that accompanies an honest identification with man and nature emanates from the heart.

All of the organs have a part in maintaining the quality and quantity of the blood, but the heart is the Emperor and therefore directs it. The small intestine is the yang organ of the heart network, which separates food and liquid into what is beneficial or harmful. After this chi can be absorbed by the spleen and incorporated into the blood, which then flows to the liver.

Heart problems are often evident in inflammatory

complaints of the small intestine.

The heart is the house of the spirit but if the heart suffers shock, great joy or sorrow then restlessness (of spirit) sleeplessness or worse can result. The memory can suffer and agitation becomes the norm.

When heart chi disperses the following symptoms become evident. The skin appears grey and lifeless, the demeanour lethargic and the extremities cold. The sufferer appears to be lost and without direction and often anxious and stressed.

The heart's emotion is joy and its nature is that of fire. The heart spreads its joy like a steadily burning flame rather than a forest fire. Excesses are not for the heart and meditation remains its finest ally.

The liver network

The liver is the general ordering his forces of chi and blood throughout the body. His energy is that of spring and new life bursting up and out with vitality and growth.

The liver stores and disperses the blood, exemplifying its yin and yang functions, and therefore facilitates the flow of chi. Anger is the emotion of the liver, an emotion that ought not to be allowed to go to extremes. If over-expressed or suppressed, damage and blockage can result. Freeflow is the essence of liver function, and many liver complaints are due to its obstruction.

In TCM the term that translates as tendons includes the idea of complete interaction between ligaments, tendons and muscles. The activity and suppleness of this system depends on liver chi and blood, as does the condition of the eyes.

The gallbladder is the paired organ of this network, and is the only yang organ, which also has a storage (yin) aspect. Bile is the substance it stores and secretes, which helps digestion and elimination.

Together, the liver and gallbladder are said to aid in clarity of thought and preparation capabilities. The expertise of the General is in his strategic skills – if these are deficient it is surely because the liver and gallbladder are not functioning in unison.

It is crucial to understand that to the TCM

practitioner, emotional difficulties are caused by misdirected or unbalanced energies. When the liver chi is blocked, it stagnates, and this manifests as frustrated energy. The freeflow of chi is the single most important ingredient in the overall balance/health of the body.

Inadequate liver performance causes stagnant chi and, ultimately, stagnant blood. If the chi is stagnant the other organs suffer loss of balance, creating anxieties, anger and stress. The glands might receive an excess of heat, causing inflammation and pain. Exhaustion is a regularly experienced result of liver chi stagnation. When liver blood stagnates it is responsible for painful muscle spasm, eye disorders and even tumours.

In emotional terms, the partnership of liver and gallbladder aids in the construction of plans, and the skills with which to actualise them. It is for this reason that the liver is called the General.

The attributes of a skilful General are clarity and vision, flexibility and strength. When these attributes are balanced, he can influence his forces in an equally healthy manner, when he is unstable, those who depend on him will exhibit instability also.

The spleen network

Representing earth in the microcosm, the spleen is at the centre. The spleen transforms the basic substance then transports the energy and nourishment, from which chi and blood are formed, throughout the body. This provides a balance, to assist in the continuity of the human organism. Despite operating in what are sometimes extreme conditions, the movement of energy and substance from one part of the body to another, assists in promoting constancy.

The spleen thus provides balance, from which comes our adaptability and resourcefulness. A healthy spleen network is essential for dealing with stress, whether its basis is emotional, mental or physical.

The spleen/stomach network governs the size and shape of the body; therefore problems in this area are usually the result of an imbalance. A healthy network will increase or diminish the transformation of substance, to blood and chi, depending on the body's need - for movement or stillness.

An unhealthy network, for instance one damaged by dampness, produces a failure to convert fluids and an excess of mucus and phlegm. This causes the conversion processes to become sluggish, creating further problems.

All of the organs have a part in producing and preserving blood: the spleen controls the blood by keeping it in the vessels. The spleen nourishes the vessel walls, but if the network is unhealthy it may not do this well. Varicose veins, haemorrhage and seepage of blood result from this kind of malfunction.

Holding its earth position, at the centre, the spleen balances the polarity of heart and kidney. It is also said to keep the other organs in place, like satellites, via a subtle gravitational energy.

Its primary emotion is thought. The clear energy of the spleen reaches the brain and allows for clarity of mind. While we may not understand how thought, or mental function, can be an emotion, it becomes easier when we think about the movement of the earth. Its motion is to continually turn. This parallels either the churning, obsessive kind of thinking that results in emotional stress, or the relaxed and open thinking that we associate with meditation.

The sixty-mile-an-hour obsessive thinking, usually created by holding on to negative energy patterns, manifests in the physical body blockages of chi. This is usually felt as a knot under the ribs, which affects the balance between the polar opposites of heart and kidney. This has an emotional manifestation, which we call fear. We can easily see how a continuation of this kind of disturbance might result in all manner of pathologies.

The stomach is the yang companion to the spleen. It requires liquid (which is yin) to perform its main function of moistening food in order to transform it. The spleen requires yang heat to balance its own dampness.

As far as their individual chi is concerned, spleen chi rises while stomach chi sinks. If these reverse for any reason, waste will not sink to the intestines and the organs and blood vessels will not maintain their correct balance. Again this produces numerous problems and diseases.

The body orifice that relates to the spleen is the mouth and its sense is taste. In TCM the five tastes also have a corresponding organ:

The heart relates to bitter

The liver to acid   The spleen to sweet

The kidney to salt   The lung to pungent

The lung network

The lungs are viewed as Ministering between the inner and outer worlds. Mixing the chi of the heaven (breath) with the chi of earth (food) is the primary activity, but equal dispensation (to the rest of the body) is important. Like the General (the liver) his function is as a mediator, but his time is autumn, and his nature that of metal (condensed essence). This is the alchemy of the Taoists, of changing that which is coarse (air and food), to essence, or chi. The lungs then expel that, which is impure and begin again. The action of the lungs depends on rhythm, on a relaxed breath. On inhalation, the movement of chi is slowed and speeds up again as the lungs inhale.

The Taoists favoured chi gung exercises to gain conscious control of the balance of chi. Through the control of the breath and chi they achieved mental, emotional and physical balance, thus making it possible to relax the heart and achieve spiritual harmony, via meditation, also.

A further function of the lungs is to condense and transmit energy down into the depths of the body.

Chi is breath, and so the lungs manage the chi of the whole system. It is the action of respiration that propels the chi throughout the body. The lungs draw in oxygen and pure chi from the surrounding air, mixing it with the food chi from the spleen. This forms zhong, or harmonious, chi and is distributed to the rest of the body. A dysfunction of the lung network causes immediate loss of energy and balance.

The condition of the nose and voice are also directly connected to the health of the lung system. Breathing difficulties, via the nose, reflect the state of the lungs and vice versa, while the strength of the voice indicates the strength of the lung chi. Posture is also an important factor determining the power of voice and quality of breath.

Sudden temperature deviations, that frequently accompany a change of season, are often blamed for health problems. This is never more obvious than in the movement from summer to autumn. During this time, when the metal element condenses and withdraws, the body is vulnerable to sudden cold snaps.

Allowing the inner movement of retreat preserves the energy, but the tendency is to ignore the warning signs. The colder months make different demands on the whole system, and these are ignored at our peril. Misery and sickness often come to us at this time of year, and this is a direct result of refusing to alter our life styles to fit the seasons.

As an extension of this idea, TCM views the skin as the third lung. When the pores are open heat, damp and cold can enter, and body chi and essence can escape. This means that if the lung chi is depleted, we are vulnerable to attack from outside sources.

When the lung chi is healthy and balanced, it is more able to control the body temperature via 涼汗 sweating and the opening and closing of the pores. When cold, damp or heat have already caused illness, the lung strategy is to expel their influences by heating the body, opening the pores and pressing them out by excess sweating.

TCM also claims that we can pick up negative emotions from other people when our resources are low.

The skin is nourished by the chi and fluid of the lungs; therefore the condition of the skin mirrors that of the lungs. When the skin is red, there is excessive heat in the lungs; too much damp and the skin is likely to be suffer from weeping sores; deficiencies often manifest as dry and flaky skin. These are some of the indications of lung problems, which the TCM practitioner can use in his/her diagnosis.

The large intestine is the yang partner in the lung network, eliminating the waste products of digestion and the metabolic processes. It is the function of this network to enable us to let go in all senses of the word. When the large intestine or the lung is functioning incorrectly, we tend to hold on to negative thoughts and emotions. This creates a spiral of negativity and illness, which can culminate in extreme behaviour syndromes.

What might manifest, in the first instance, as clinging behaviour patterns, triggers the desire for freedom. This then becomes the opposite extreme in which we exhibit a total lack of control. The next step is a re-emergence of the desire for self-discipline and inhibitive behaviour again takes over.

A return to health is seen when we re-establish healthy extremes. In the case of the lung network, these are signified by the limits of inhalation and exhalation. With the breathing exercises of chi gung, yin and yang are directed and balanced throughout the organism, thereby giving form to the farthest extensions of the physical and ethereal bodies.

The emotion of the lung is grief. When we must let go of things that have been important to our development, we naturally experience sorrow. An excess of this emotion causes an excess of inward movement. The chest becomes concave, causing restriction of the heart and lungs.

The kidney network

The important thing to know about the kidneys is that they store jing or essence. Jing is the most refined material of the human organism. In some texts, we are told that jing is irreplaceable, that when it has been used, we die. Others suggest that the Taoist alchemists knew how to both preserve and increase the amount of jing. Whichever is true, it is certain that without it there is no growth or development. Chi gung and T'ai chi are both said to preserve and increase the quality of this vital substance.

This substance is the essential basis from which all of our tissues are formed. Kidney jing produces Marrow, which TCM practitioners view as the primary component of bone, bone marrow, the spinal cord and the construction of the physical brain. A deficiency of kidney jing causes many of the problems common to these areas.

Taoist sexual alchemy is becoming increasingly prominent in the West, and many claim to achieve greater and more enriching relationships as a result of these practises. They are also reported to result in a perfect balance of the Three Treasures (see above). As we have said, the jing, chi and shen are the foundation of all energy adjustments and conversions throughout the body. They are separate only in our conceptions of them; in reality they are mutually dependent.

The interaction of jing (primary essence) and shen (spirit) are the yin and yang: the heaven and earth within the human form. The movement of Chi, via the meridians, makes this possible. Chi is the mediator, the spark providing a linkage between that which is above and that which is below.

In TCM the process is of aiding, rather than impeding, the conservation of kidney jing. This is so that chi is generated and balanced, in a manner that allows for a healthy expression of the spirit. This is perceived as true harmony – the correct interaction of the Three Treasures, and the whole organism.

Kidney chi sustains the reproductive organs, and difficulties arising in these areas, is often as a result of the excessive use of jing. For a man, excessive sex in early years engenders a lack of vitality later; just as for a woman too many children will give the same result.

Kidney essence is responsible for maturation, in that bone marrow and calcium, red blood cells, hair and teeth are under its control. The physical is called the sea of marrow, and the kidney chi is responsible for its quality of function.

The ear is the orifice of the kidney and as we age, and suffer a depletion of jing, we also suffer the onset of hearing difficulties.

A further vital function of the kidneys is that of controlling the liquids of the body. The yang element controls balance and distribution, while kidney yin provides the source for all body fluids. Sexual juices, tears, sweat, saliva, spinal fluid, mucus, urine and other secretions of the body originate from the fusion of yin essence that we obtain via food and breath, and the jing of our parents.

Deficiency of kidney yang allows for an excess of kidney yin, which creates difficulties throughout the body. Kidney yang warms the whole body, enlivens both spleen and liver, and activates the shen of the heart. When there is a deficiency, these functions, and many more, do not receive the initial spark of energy they require to kick-start their activity. The body suffers cold; breath and digestion begin to fail; waste is not filtered correctly; reproductive and hearing problems occur.

Excessive use of drugs, alcohol, sex, strong tastes or sleeplessness and overwork, all place a great strain on the kidneys.

The bladder is the yang organ in the kidney network, and deals directly with the waste liquids. Between them they control the cycle of conversion, re-assimilation and emission.

A part of the bladder meridian divides down both sides of the spine, and it is via this meridian that all of the other internal organs have their primary treatment points.

Fear is the kidney's emotion: simple, basic, animal fear. At its most extreme, this kind of fear can cause an immediate loss of waste. It is a survival technique, linked to the unknown, to the dark night and coldest winter. It is on the one hand an instinctive, uncontrollable urge, and on the other it is the base from which we become worldly wise.

Knowledge and understanding of our true worldly situation, brings a balanced acceptance of our individual strengths and weaknesses. From this acceptance comes the desire for personal improvement. Such personal growth must itself be based on the true nature of the human condition.

Chinese philosophy, psychology and all things medical are founded on this viable form of self-development. The I Ching contains 64 hexagrams, each of which is made up of six changing lines. It is a complex form of study and understanding of the human, worldly and cosmic condition. At its base, however, just as in TCM, it is simply the theory of yin and yang.

The I Ching and TCM both follow the Chinese holistic viewpoint: that two forces, principles or archetypes generate all things. These forces (yin and yang) represent the polar expressions of the One: that which cannot be named or described – the Tao.

When yang is full, it becomes yin, and vice versa.

The sanjiao and pericardium and pulse

The five organ networks above have Western equivalents, but the sanjiao (triple heater) and pericardium (heart protector) have no Western counterparts.

Nevertheless, an understanding of TCM would be incomplete without some mention of them, and so we will give a brief description.

The pericardium is simply the protective outer covering of the heart. Its protection is primarily against yang (heat) energies, in the form of fevers, which it confines within itself, restricting its passage to the heart.

The sanjiao synchronizes the movement, transformation and function of water in the three (san) areas of the body (jiao). These are the chest and upper and lower abdomen. The sanjiao also controls the temperature of the body, by aiding in the transfer of chi.

The method for taking the pulse, favoured by TCM practitioners, using three fingers, measures the energy of these three centres, and therefore the condition of their related organ networks.

The fingers press along the radial artery on one wrist, then the other. The index finger (closest to the wrist) refers to the upper burner, the middle to the middle burner and the ring finger to the lower burner. The practitioner is testing the pulse rate, strength and rhythm in order to diagnose the constancy of the chi and blood flow, to and from the internal organs.

Pulses are taken on both wrists as each has different organs in relationship to it. These are as follows:

Left hand:	Index finger	= heart
	Middle finger	= liver
	Ring finger	= kidney yin
Right hand:	Index finger	= lung
	Middle finger	= spleen
	Ring finger	= kidney yang

The practitioner uses three pressures – superficial, middle and deep. There is a subtle art in diagnosis via the pulse, in Chinese medicine: an art, which can only be learned by constant practise.

The following list is in no way comprehensive, as it is the purpose of this book to offer only a simple insight into TCM. We do hope, however, that it will aid the beginner in understanding the intricacy of some of its components.

A floating pulse indicates an attack by cold, wind or heat.

If floating and fast, resistance from the chi is indicated.

Rapid pulse is an excess of internal heat.

Slow pulse indicates excessive cold.

Pulses without energy suggest deficiency of chi and blood.

Weak pulses are usually yin disorders, while strong pulses indicate yang.

An irregular pulse often implies heart problems.

It should be remembered that, while an excess of yang generates heat, it could also derive from insufficient yin.

Obviously there is much more to pulse analysis than we have presented, but the above is enough to demonstrate its complexity. We will return to our brief examination of the triple burner.

The upper burner encloses the heart and lungs and is responsible for transforming breath into energy. The lung controls chi and the heart governs blood.

The heartbeat keeps pace with the breath and the chi and blood flow together. When these do not function in unison many difficulties become manifest. An obstruction in the flow of lung chi creates a blockage in blood circulation followed by heart problems. Heart problems cause difficulties with the breath, and so on.

The middle burner houses the spleen and liver and transmutes energy from food. It must then transmit the energy around the body. Blockages in this centre make it difficult for the higher and lower centres to interact.

In the lower burner the energy contributed by our

parents, (original jing) validates the potential of the other centres to transmute their energies. Here the kidneys, bladder and intestines are housed, and the energy produced concerns fertility, development and maturation.

CHAPTER 5

The Eight Patterns or Guiding Principles and Five Phase Theory

These are simply one way of arranging information received during examination. They are, in fact, a system of four pairs of polar qualities, designed to organise and classify indications of disharmony. They are paired as follows:

- Yin/yang
- Heat/cold
- Excess/deficiency
- Inside/outside

Yin and yang divides the other three pairs as follows:

- Hot/excess/outside are yang.
- Cold/deficiency/inside are yin.

- Heat/cold define the energy balance.
- Excess/deficiency defines strength of disease versus strength of organism.

- Exterior/interior defines the location of the problem.

In reality, the last three pairs subordinate to the first – yin/yang. Remember that the primary function of TCM analysis is to judge whether the problem indicates predominance if yin or yang.

By using this simple method of summarising his readings, the practitioner can establish the condition, disposition and location of the chi, blood and fluids of the body, as well as in relation to the organs.

The use of the eight principles is as a guide only, and the practitioner will tend to be flexible with their use. Patterns can change swiftly as a malady goes through its various stages, and these must be mapped in order that the correct medication is prescribed.

Finally in this chapter, we will take a brief look at the Extraordinary Fu organs. They are the brain, bone, Marrow, uterus, blood vessels and gall bladder. Like the fu organs, they are deemed to be hollow but their function is more like that of the zang organs. They store jing, blood and marrow and function as follows:

The brain is called the sea of marrow, as this is where it is stored.

The bones of course, store bone marrow.

Marrow supplies the bone and brain with nourishment.

The uterus controls menstruation and conception.
Blood vessels hold the blood.
The gall bladder stores bile.

The five emotions and the five outside evils (climates)

These are:
- Emotions – anger, joy, pensiveness, sorrow, and fear/fright.
- Climates – cold, wind, heat, damp, dryness/summer heat.

Both of these groups correspond to the five elements (five phase theory). We will add them to our river map diagram, in order that we can observe how they interact.

Summer
Fire/heat/joy

Spring   **Late summer**
wood/wind/anger   **Earth/dampness/pensive**

Winter   **Autumn**
Water/cold/fear   **Metal/dryness/grief**

Their interaction is best demonstrated by the sheng and ke cycles. Sheng means mutual support and ke, means mutual control.

The supporting sequence is as follows:

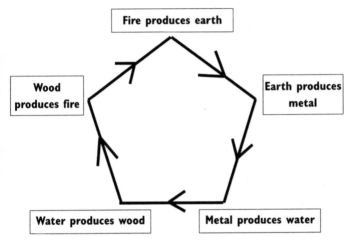

The controlling sequence is as follows:

Fire controls metal

Wood controls earth

Earth controls water

Water controls fire

Metal controls wood

The five elements, or phases, interact consistent with patterns of generation and control. The ke cycle (mutual control) refers to the manner that the elements control each other via the dynamic of restraint. The sheng cycle (mutual generation) indicates the support sequence of the five elements.

The five-phase theory is the Chinese view of how balance is achieved. The control cycle creates limits, while the generating cycle promotes expansion. This can be simply demonstrated as follows:

Fire controls metal (via melting) – earth supports metal (creates minerals).

Earth controls water (blocking and inhibiting) – metal supports water (via refined materials).

Metal controls wood (cutting) – water supports wood (nourishment).

Water controls fire (extinguishes) – wood generates fire (as fuel).

Fire supports earth (reducing wood to ash) – wood controls earth (covering).

By using the shen and ke cycles for the organ networks and their attributes, we can observe the simplicity of the five-phase methodology.

A practical example of this system might be:

Fire promotes earth – therefore the heart supports the spleen by contributing heat and blood, necessary for the digestion of food. Conversely, wood controls earth, so the chi of the liver controls (stimulates) the ability of the spleen to transform food.

The five-phase methodology is meant to simplify the interaction between the organ networks and their processes. Where one network is overly controlled, or generated with an excess of energy by another network, it suffers because of that excess or deficiency. On the one hand it cannot support or control those networks, which depend on it, on the other produces, in its turn, an excess of energy or control. We need only create a simple example as follows:

If the liver is suffering excess, first the spleen then the kidney are involved. This will continue until all networks have succumbed, and the whole organism is contaminated.

Should the energy of the liver be insufficient, the deficiency follows the same pathway as above resulting in an overall inability to function.

CHAPTER 6
Acupuncture

The system of meridians (channels vessels)

The subtle energy system of TCM is something akin
to magic for most of us in the West. The idea that
energy travels around the body in channels moving in
precise patterns, appearing and disappearing at
specific locations, is difficult to accept. Not because
we in the West have no imagination, or are intolerant
to new ideas, but simply because these channels
cannot be seen. Their actuality has not been proved.

Our Western system of physiology and anatomy is
based on verifiable data, demonstrations of physical
presence. When something new does not fit into our
system of categories and scientific confirmation, we
know to be sceptical, and rightly so. There are more
charlatans than there are Shamans, in every field of
study. But isn't it that the concept threatens us?

The idea that a system exists, through which every
individual might understand the nature of all things,

know his/her place in the cosmos and be responsible for his/her own health and well-being, is quite daunting. But it is only so if we presume that either that system, or our own, is correct. Because of course both systems have proved their viability. They both work.

Perhaps the differences lie only in the point of view. Science and the social order surrounding it, appears to originate in the clear thinking mind. To understand the nature and relation of things, and how this might aid in individual development, requires an intuitive and receptive mind.

This is the yin and yang of it. A consolidation of these mental attributes, of these viewpoints, offers a balanced structure, a synthesis of primary characteristics.

With such an attitude we can fully exploit the Chinese approach to health and balance. When we begin to use this system, especially where it touches on the channels or meridians, we can only do so with a receptive frame of mind. If it shows results, we need only accept that it does so. We are not required to accept the whole system. In this way we can practise using the receptive skills of our minds, and in doing so, awakening our intuitive attributes.

There are many analogies we might use for our initial conception. We can view them in ways we are used to, as arrangements that parallel our nervous systems, as structures similar to the network of veins or even like a system of canals or rivers. The problem with such an analogy is that we can easily forget that we are using a metaphor. To awaken our receptive and intuitive skills, we need to move a little further from our safe and sensible thinking.

The organ networks of TCM communicate at a subtle energy level. Chi and blood, shen and jing, are basically energetic materials, providing the motive force for all of those networks. The physical body demonstrates optimum health or otherwise, depending on the support of these dynamic properties. But we must remember that health is only a symptom or manifestation of these primary energies.

The invisible chi travels around the body along a system of channels, as well as through the blood. There are twelve primary chi channels and eight extraordinary meridians. Along these channels are acupuncture points known as men, which means gate. These are analogous to the city gates of feudal times, which were opened only to admit friendly forces. The men are to be found in small depressions of the skin, the opening and closing of which, alters the dynamics of blood and chi flow.

The insertion of thin, stainless steel needles into these points, are used to either stimulate or restrain the circulation of energy. This disturbance of the flow one way or the other has significant effects on the physical body.

The needles are inserted to a depth of a fraction of an inch to a few inches, creating a variety of sensations. These sensations, from minor tingling to soreness, from discomfort to an almost painful pressure, are manifestations or symptoms of the presence of chi. Thus the evidence of chi might be near to or far from the initial insertion point. This, TCM practitioners tell us, substantiates the existence of channels.

The channels, as we have stated, correspond to the five organ networks. There is a sixth, the pericardium, which functions as a yin organ whose corresponding yang organ is the sanjiao.

We will repeat the organ networks once more, with the yin organ first:

The heart network includes the small intestine.

The lung network includes the large intestine.

The pericardium and the sanjiao go together.

As does the liver and gallbladder.

And the kidney and bladder.

Finally the spleen and stomach are paired.

There are six paired yin and yang channels – three on the arm, three on the leg, correspondingly.

Thus we have, with abbreviations:

The heart channel of hand shaoyin.	**He**
The small intestine channel of hand taiyang.	**SI**
The lung channel of hand taiyin.	**L**
The large intestine channel of hand yangming.	**LI**
The pericardium channel of hand jueyin.	**Per**
The sanjiao channel of hand shaoyang.	**San**
The liver channel of foot jueyin.	**Li**
The gall bladder channel of foot shaoyang.	**GB**
The kidney channel of foot shaoyin.	**K**
The bladder channel of foot taiyang.	**Bl**
The spleen channel of foot taiyin.	**S**
The stomach channel of foot yangming.	**St**

The flow of energy through the twelve meridians is as follows:

The three yin arm channels (**He, L, Per**) flow from the area of the upper burner, along the arms to the hands, and merge with the three yang channels (**LI, SI, San**), then travel to the head.

There they merge with the equivalent leg yang channels (**GB, Bl, St**), and sink to the feet, where they merge with the yin leg channels of (**Li, S, K**), then returning to the upper burner, completing the cycle.

The eight extraordinary channels

The chi jing ba mai are the strange or mysterious
meridians of TCM. They were discovered about two
thousand years ago, but not a great deal is known of
them. There is some research on them, mostly in
Japan, but the theories and results of such research
are inconsistent. We will look at what is generally
understood to be their primary functions, both
practically and esoterically.

They are:
• The governing vessel called – du mai.
• The conception vessel called – ren mai.
• Thrusting vessel or chong mai.
• Girdle vessel or dai mai.
• The yang heel vessel called yangchiao mai.
• The yin heel vessel called yinchiao.
• Finally the yang linking vessel – the yangwei mai
• And the yin linking vessel – the yinwei mai.

Their known primary functions are as follows:
I That they constitute reservoirs for the twelve
   organ networks.
       They absorb excess chi from the networks
   replacing it when there is a deficit. Acupuncture
   needles 'open' the gates of these reservoirs. These
   gates, or men as they are called, regulate the
   concentration of flow and volume of chi in the

reservoirs.

When we experience trauma, there will be a deficit of chi in one or more of the networks. The organs and their dependent structures will then suffer stress and eventual damage, unless they receive the chi that they need to restore balance. The reservoirs automatically release energy to restore the status quo, thus preventing long-term problems.

2   The governing, conception and thrusting vessels act as protectors from external attack. They are responsible for the circulation of the wei chi (protective chi).

3   They circulate essence or jing chi across the trunk. They convey it to the blood system, liver network, bone marrow, uterus and brain and spinal chord.

4   The conception and thrusting vessels are said to regulate the life cycles – in men these cycles occur every eight years, in women every seven.

5   They form the basis of many chi gong and meditation exercises. The eight vessels are seen to be more primordial than the twelve, balancing the extremes of yin/yang, interior/exterior, left/right and above/below. On one level they are perceived as the organisers of the original embryo, from conception to birth. On another level they represent the ideal energy interchange between heaven and earth.

They correspond to the eight trigrams of the I

Ching, which symbolize the total number of
energy phenomenon possible, in the cosmos, the
world and man.

The primary chi gong exercise for the conception
and governor vessels is called the 'small circulation
exercise'. This entails filling both vessels with chi,
which is then circulated. As a part of this chi flow, the
kidney essence will have been transmuted into chi,
and the brain, spinal chord and shen (spirit), will
have received nourishment.

Only the first two of the eight meridians have
specific acupuncture points. The conception and
governor vessels both have pathways and
acupuncture points, and both originate in the middle
of the belly. The du mai, the governor vessel, follows
the centre of the back, the ren mai, the conception
vessel follows the centre front.

The embryonic breathing of the Taoists recalls the
symmetry of pre-birth. The front is concave, soft and
yin, the back is hard convex and yang.

The governor vessel at the back is described as,
'the sea of yang channels', and as its name suggests, it
governs all yang channels.

The conception channel is at the front and
associated with yin, blood and form. It is responsible
for the building of new life, whether through the
bearing of children, transforming food and drink or
the renewal of life via an interchange of yang with the
governor vessel.

The pathway of the governor vessel (the du mai)

The meaning of du mai includes the idea of capacity to rule. The du mai is the yang meridian, which flows up the back of the body. It begins in the lower tan tien, (the lower stomach) and surfaces in the perineum. From there it follows the spine to the back of the head, where it enters the brain. It then flows over the head to the centre of the forehead and then to the roof of the mouth.

We can look at some of the major points along this meridian in order to gain a better understanding of the Chinese perception of chi circulation. We will also investigate some of the treatments at these points.

Governor vessel 1 (chang chiang)

Location: between coccyx and anus

The name is translated as long and strong, with the idea of stability. The character for strength, chiang, includes the symbol of a bow. The idea is that the bow contains the energy by which the arrow can be released to great distance. If the base of the spine is stable, yang energy travels directly to the brain, creating clarity of thought sound vision. During chi gong exercises, it is recommended that the muscles at this point be contracted, allowing the chi to circulate freely.

Problems of lower back pain and lumbago can be eased at this point. Also problems as diverse as piles, enteritis and proctoptosis.

Governor vessel 4 (ming men)
Location: between second and third lumbar vertebrae
The name of this point means, the gate of life, and is
linked with the energy of the kidneys. Arguably the
most important point on the body, it is the
connection between inherited energies and the
capacity to convert them, thereby fulfilling
potentiality. It connects our foundation and our
development. Often depicted as a cauldron in which
the essence of the kidneys is heated by the fire of
kidney yang.

This point is used to strengthen the kidneys,
encourage energy production and warm and energize
the whole body. It can also help to relieve headaches,
back problems and difficulties of the reproductive
area.

Governor vessel 14 (da zhui)
*Location: back of the neck between 7th cervical and 1st
thoracic vertebrae*
The translation of the name is great hammer and
refers to the protrusion of the bones. At this point all
of the yang meridians merge and its main use is the
passage of energy between head and back. Work at
this point relieves colds, fevers and bronchial
problems. Neck, shoulder and back difficulties as well
as some psychosis' can all be alleviated at this point.

Governor vessel 16 (feng fu)

Location: middle of the neck at the base of the skull

Here the governor vessel enters the brain, creating the clarity of thought and vision we mentioned at the base point of this meridian. There are many simple chi gung exercises, developed to keep this area loose and relaxed, thereby preventing tension and confused thinking. Also useful for relieving headaches and mental pressure. Care should be taken to obstruct cold and wind from entering the head, as these are primary causes of headaches.

Governor vessel 20 (bai hui)

Location: top of the head between the line of the ears

The governor vessel merges with the six yang meridians at this point. In tai chi we begin the form by visualising the suspension of the body by a silver cord, from this point. Another of the primary points of the body, work at this point aids in resuscitation after breakdowns or unconsciousness. Can be used to relieve headaches, help with memory problems, and reduce blood pressure.

Yintang (no number for this point)

Location: between the eyebrows

This is the upper tan tien, also called the brow chakra. Not too important in medical terms, but used in the chi gung exercises. Is occasionally recommended, in tui na, for relieving headaches.

Governor vessel 28

Location: between the top lip and teeth, the yin jiao, or
'yin crossing' is the place where the governor and
conception vessels meet. During chi gung and t'ai chi
the tongue is pressed gently to the roof of the mouth,
in order that the chi can circulate. The yang of the
governing vessel and the yin of the conception vessel
are then connected. The nose is the 'gate of heaven'
(yang), and the mouth is the 'door of the earth' (yin),
and these are also connected as a result of this
circulation.

The connecting of the rear meridian to the front
meridian at the position of governor 28, brings us to
the point in the cleft of the chin. This point is:
Conception 24 It is used primarily for mouth and
facial problems.

Conception vessel 22 (Tiantu)

*Location: the hollow at the base of the neck, just above the
breastbone*
Known as the 'sea of yin meridians', this point is
where the cooling yin energy gains access to the head.
The throat and brain are moistened by the fertile
essences, which also achieve entrance to the head via
this area. The point is used to relieve throat
difficulties in a general way.

Conception vessel 17 (tanzhong)

Location: on the breastbone, on the line of the nipples

Another of the primary points of the body, the tan zhong (the higher sea of chi), is responsible for much of the body's harmony. The various rhythms and cycles are governed by the breath, and include such diverse behaviour as the movement of food, heartbeat action of the pores. More importantly the chi and blood is controlled from this area. Chi gung teaches us to gain conscious control of our rhythms and cycles, by controlling the breathing rhythms while observing the circulations. Work at this point helps with heart and chest pain, as well as lung difficulties.

The centre where inherited chi gathers the rest of the chi to insure that the body conforms to the required patterns.

Conception vessel 12 (zhong wan)

Location: four inches above the navel

This centre relates to the spleen and stomach, correcting problems at this level, and governing the energy input and distribution from our food and drink. Difficulties dealt with at this point include, blood pressure, vomiting and other digestion problems.

Conception vessel 6 (qihai)

Location: an inch and a half below the navel

Translated as 'the sea of chi' this point the yin and

yang mix together, drawing the fire of 'the gate of life' to excite and energise blood and body fluids. This point and the next, vessel 4, are important for increasing the flow of energy and are constantly used in concentration and meditation techniques. Used generally for abdominal problems and specifically for menstruation difficulties in women.

Conception vessel 4 (guanyuan)
Location: three inches below the navel
The 'gateway to the origins' merges with the yin meridians of spleen, kidneys and liver, as well as connecting with the 'gate of life' (ming men, governor vessel 4). Here, the circulation technique begins and ends; the visualisation of movement of energy from front to back (Chen style t'ai chi) is harmonised, and the balancing and strengthening of blood and chi, with the help of conception 6, is centred.

Conception vessel I (hui yin)
Location: between the anus and scrotum (in men), or the anus and vagina (in women), the 'yin meeting' point merges with the governor vessel.
Used in chi gung to transmute energies, and in meditation/breath exercises as a starting point for circulatory visualisations. The muscles are often tensed in this area prior to these exercises (and often held throughout) in order that the chi flows freely. It is suggested, by Dr.Yee, that this is similar to pressing

the tongue to the roof of the mouth to ensure the
connection between governor and conception vessels.
Used for sexual problems, but primarily for fastening
and grounding the yang energy.

The governor vessel connects the three energy centres
(lower, middle and upper tantien). When the channel
is free of blockages the yang energy is free to enliven
the abdomen and brain, providing a harmony of
health and clarity. The conception vessel flows up the
centre front of the body, also connecting the three
centres, providing nourishment, and moist, cooling
elements to the body and brain.

There are six more of these extraordinary meridians
and we will give a brief description of each:

Chong Mai (penetrating or thrusting vessel)
The penetrating vessel is so called because its energy
moves with dynamic force. It starts at the same place
as the first two, in the lower abdomen. Then, from
slightly above the pubic bone, it travels down the legs
to the bottom of the foot. It travels upwards also,
internally, along the spinal column, encircling the area
of the mouth.

It combines yin and yang in order to produce this
explosion of creative energy. It is used to remove
stagnation of blood and chi, relieve leg pain and
reduce inflammation. Energy is provided in a

dynamic fashion when blocks have been removed.

It supports the conception vessel, and their combined chi efficiently governs that of the kidney channel. Remember that the kidneys play a vital part in mental and physical growth. Kidney essence gives rise to the marrow, which engenders spinal chord, blood and bone. When this essence is in abundance we secure health and clarity of mind, when deficient we suffer all manner of pathologies.

The thrusting vessel plays an important role in the chi gong exercise known as 'marrow washing'. The purpose of the exercise is to lead the chi to the brain via the marrow. Marrow washing uses the water path, thereby cooling excessive yang chi after which it nourishes the brain and strengthens the shen (spirit).

The girdle vessel (dai mai)

All of the meridians travel in the direction of high to low or low to high, except this one. The girdle vessel is what its name describes: a girdle of energy around the waist area, holding the other meridians in place. It passes through the 'gate of life' at the back, and 'the gate of origin' in the front. The belt of energy is meant to have a particular tension. If loose, body fluids tend to accumulate in the area of the lower burner. Excess tension produces a rigidity of movement, emotion and thought patterns.

Primarily, the girdle vessel regulates the chi of the gall bladder and circulates chi around the kidneys.

As this is all in the area of the lower tantien, the waist must be strong and relaxed in order that the chi can settle here.

The heel vessels of yin chiao mai (yang chiao mai)
The chiao mai begins at the heel, and then separates to the inside of the ankle (yin) and the outside (yang). The yin tract travels upward, passed the genital area through the centre body to the throat and eye. The yang tract travels up the back, along the shoulders to the throat and eye, where it meets the yin tract. From here it changes direction to the back of the head.

These two vessels provide harmony between primary energies, and alter the body's natural rhythms. Whenever the body is no longer in tune with rhythms of day and night, summer and winter, these channels adjust the balance. Practitioners of tui-na emphasise these vessels for the restoration of balance between fire and water, yin and yang and blood and chi.

The linking vessels of yin wei mai (yang wei mai)
These two vessels are unconnected, beginning and ending at different points. The yin channel begins inside the lower part of the calf, and then travels up the body to the throat. The yang wei begins at the outside of the foot, above the little toe, follows the outside of the leg to the head. It then travels around

the ear to back of the head. The yang channel provides much of the chi for the normal function of the muscles and protection from the five evils, whereas the yin channel protects from the five emotions. Yang wei mai defends the outside and yin wei mai, the inside.

The yang channel links with the yang meridians of the stomach, gall-bladder, bladder, triple burner and small intestine.

The yin channel links liver, kidney and spleen meridians.

We can now build a picture of the eight extraordinary vessels via their known functions. It should be remembered that energy can flow along these meridians in either direction.

The conception channel and governor channel, begin at the same point, in the middle of the abdomen. This area holds the greatest amount of yin energy.

The conception channel travels up the front of the body, the governor vessel up the spine. Between them they create a cycle of energy around the body, the conception channel being perceived as protector of original yin, the governor as director of original yang.

`These two represent the first of the ba-gua or eight trigrams of the I Ching: the energy of the conception vessel is that of k'un (primary yin/earth), the governor is chien (primary yang/heaven). Their energy is defined as contracting (yin) and expanding (yang). This means that the yin of the conception vessel helps the body to bend and protect the centre, while the governor vessel provides the energy to expand the spine and drive the body forward.

The penetrating vessel begins at the same point as the first two. It unites yin and yang forcefully, like an explosion of pent up energy creating speedy growth. The girdle vessel is like a belt around the middle of the body, holding the others in place. Its energy constantly moving, its affect is like the wind, everywhere at once, holding everything in place.

The heel vessels govern the bodily rhythms and the circulation of yin and yang through the other vessels, providing a sense of spatial balance. The linking vessels connect and control the chi and blood.

These eight vessels formulate the foundation from which the twelve other meridians function, together and with their associated organs.

We have tried to conceptualise the channels that transport the chi throughout the body. Like all the other pathways in the body i.e. the veins and the nervous system, they cover the entire organism, providing energy where required. Nevertheless it would be erroneous to view this network in the way that we perceive the networks of blood and nerves. The meridians (vessels, channels) describe an energetic process, a dynamic process that empowers all of the physical processes of the organism.

Remember that in TCM, and indeed Chinese philosophy, the belief is that Chi pervades everything in the universe. Everything is a manifestation of chi. Therefore, when we speak of channels; we mean areas in which there is a greater accumulation of this energy prospect than others. Should the dynamic flow of this energy be blocked, the physical structure will begin to break down. We call this breakdown, disease.

The acupuncture points are simply areas in which we can control the effects of the chi flow. They have been described in many ways, always metaphorically, as access points; knots in string; energy vortexes; and many more. In whatever way we conceptualise them, what they do is to alter the movement of chi. This has consequential affects on the physical organism, as we have already described.

When we apply a needle to these points, we effectively alter the pattern of energy.

Let us see what this means, in a general way, regarding treatment via acupuncture.

TCM is not magic, though its effects might seem so to the uninitiated. Treatment for headache will be more forthcoming than pain resulting from brain tumours. Some disorders might require greater lengths of time to balance than others and in some cases, as with all treatments, the condition has deteriorated so badly that there will be no full recovery at all. The process for treatment is as follows.

The practitioner, after careful analysis, chooses the point or points, to be needled. These insertions may require some manipulation or they may not. The manipulations might include rotation, pushing (with or without force), lifting slowly or swiftly, and even the use of extremely small amounts of electrical energy.

The amount of treatments, and their occurrence, varies greatly and will depend on many different factors. It should be stated and re-stated that these factors will depend themselves on the competency of the practitioner. If the reader intends to use this or any other book to attempt his own treatment, he/she should first look up the word competency in the dictionary.

However if he/she really wishes to know more about TCM with the idea of becoming a practitioner themselves, then there are many bona-fide teachers and organizations to aid them in this desire.

When we apply the term treatment to acupuncture, we are really talking about a re-balancing of energies.

When the organism is suffering from excess or deficiency, then the insertion needles is meant to reduce or increase the flow of chi. If there is too much heat or yang, the insertion should reduce the heat and/or increase the yin, cooling energy. Too much cold and the opposite is sought.

This makes the whole procedure appear really simple: just place this needle here, adjust the balance, and hey presto. Some ailments might be just so, but the likelihood is that the whole problem is much more complex.

The acupuncturist must first analyse the symptoms so that that he/she can determine the origin of the disorder. Once this understanding has been reached the root can be removed, followed by those difficulties created by the original problem, and so on.

The primary aim, of course, of all treatments must be to re-establish the balance of the primary energies.

We will now move on to the Chinese form of massage and manipulation known as tui-na.

CHAPTER 7
Tui-Na

Tui is pushing, Na is grasping.

Tui Na has been used in China for at least two thousand years, and like acupuncture and acupressure it utilizes the meridian theory. It practises a variety of massage and manipulation techniques to restore a balanced flow of chi throughout the body, thereby re-establishing a state of optimum health.

At the foundation of its vast array of techniques are acupressure techniques to stimulate the flow of chi in a direct manner, manipulation techniques to establish a realignment of the muscle and ligament relationships, and massage of the muscle and tendons. Tui Na also includes the use of herbs and potions to aid in the healing of tissue and bone, and cupping and moxibustion techniques.

There are many different schools working under the Tui Na umbrella. All of their methods encompass the basic techniques but focus on one particular aspect.

There is the Nei Gung school whose methods are centred on Nei Gung (also known as chi gung) exercises and particular massage techniques, which allow the immediate release of healing energies. The Bone Setting School specializes in injuries to joints and the nervous system, while the Single Finger school emphasizes the internal healing and the use of acupressure techniques. Another of the better-known systems is the Rolling method school that focus mainly on muscle and tendon techniques. Other schools emphasize pain relief and the relief of strain and trigger release techniques.

It is not our intention to teach in this simple primer, only to provide an overview of TCM. Nevertheless we feel it might be helpful to describe the basic use of the following techniques as if the reader were performing the session.

A session of Tui Na involves an analysis of the difficulty, which will include history, environment and diet. The history will focus on that of the particular problem but, as in all Chinese healing therapies, will include the patient's background as well. Observation and intuition are of primary importance at this stage of the session. The practitioner will have made certain observations already by watching the patient's movements. Was there any imbalance, movement toward or away from the centre? While questioning the patient about the condition he/she will check skin tone and the general condition of the face.

Tui Na will deal primarily with external (physical problems) rather than internal (Chi deficiencies) maladies, but other of its aspects includes these also, so it is necessary to broaden the diagnosis.

It is important that the patient be relaxed in the session, so the massage and manipulation techniques described in this chapter will require practise. It is necessary that the patient be confident in the your ability and comfortable in his surroundings, so preparation is important.

The simplest way to practise the massage strokes and various manipulations is to practise on yourself. Make the movements even and smooth, pressing deep into the muscle for the most thorough effect. Rhythm of movement is essential and should be carried out with your arms and hands as relaxed as possible. If you intend serious practise of the Oriental healing arts I would suggest that you take up one of the internal martial arts such as T'ai Chi and/or find a competent teacher of one or all aspects of TCM.

As your skills increase you might practise on your partner, friends or family, noting which strokes and manipulations work the best and in which areas. You might also observe that various amounts of pressure work with different people. Young or strong people can cope with an intensity of pressure and fast flowing movements that older or weaker people could not.

Remember always that the movements should be

even and thorough but never rough.

As with most sessions of this type begin with the head and work down, front of the body first, finishing with the back. However this is not written in stone, so always use intuition. Use a massage table if possible so it is easy to reach your entire patient, while not being tiring to you. If the healing is specific and you are dealing with one area only it will do no harm to relax the patient first with some simple massage in the surrounding areas of the problem. Obviously do not do so if this will cause pain or discomfort.

At this point you should note the two kinds of massage: these are centripetal and centrifugal. The first means simply that the blood is massaged toward the heart speeding the return of blood and lymph, and the latter means away from the heart. Centripetal is also an aid in dispersing chi and blood stagnation.

In the next section we will look at the various techniques to be used, and some of the areas in which they might apply. It must be understood that intuition is of primary importance, and that while these techniques apply in some areas better than others, a Tui Na session is about the individual. In all Chinese healing methods this paradigm applies. Firstly we will look at some of the simple massage techniques that we can apply ourselves.

For the session find a warm relaxing place, where you can wear as few clothes as possible. Shorts and Tshirt are fine. The sessions ought to be fairly regular and need last no more than twenty minutes. Apart from general health aspects, you will gain a direct understanding of how your body works, as well as first hand knowledge of the individual benefits of each technique.

Preparation: rub the hands together 30 times, vigorously, before each exercise.

The foot

For these techniques we need to be fairly loose and
relaxed. Pull the foot up and using the palm, press up
and down the sole. Do this 25 times each foot. This
will directly improve circulation of blood and chi,
reduce blood pressure and benefit the brain.

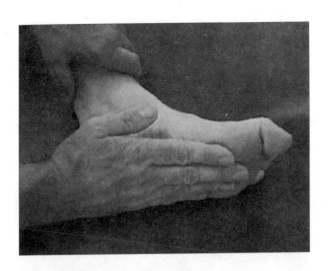

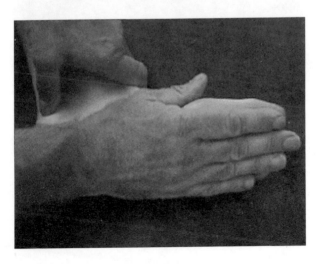

The legs

With the thumb and forefinger, press into the depressions below the knees using circular movements, while rolling the body-weight forward and back. Repeat 25 times .

Benefits are for reducing leg and stomach pain, preventing arthritis and improving digestion.

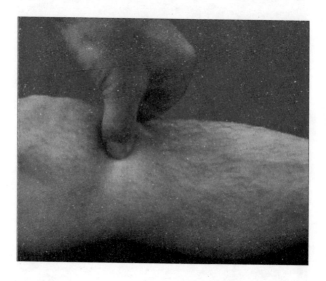

This next exercise increases the flow of blood and chi through the six foot-meridians. Press down each leg from thigh to ankle and back up again.

Repeat the exercise 30 or more times, then relax for a minute or so.

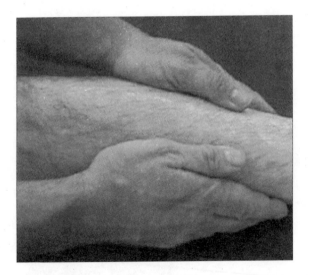

The back

After rubbing the hands vigorously, place them immediately in the area of the kidneys. Rub up and down about 40 times then relax the arms. If you have experienced pain or discomfort in this area, repeat the exercise when the arms are relaxed. If this or any other difficulty persists be sure to visit a medical practitioner.

Benefits the kidneys, and therefore all other organs indirectly. It reduces back pain and helps prevent problems occurring in the genital area.

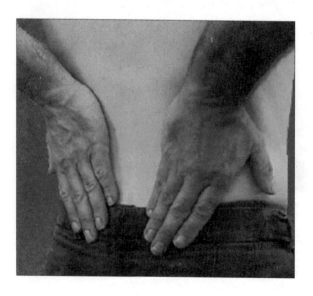

The arms

Hold your hands in the prayer position and rub them together vigorously. The six hand-channels, and therefore their respective organs, all benefit from this exercise. (Use this exercise prior to the other techniques)

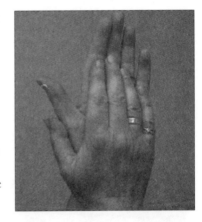

Press and rub the arms from shoulder to wrist, and back again, in the same way as for the legs. Do the same for the back of the arm as the front. Repeat each sequence about 30 times. Again this increases the flow of chi/blood.

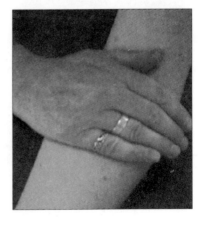

Front of the body

Press and squeeze the muscles of the chest, one side at a time, and moving in toward the breastbone. Then make circular motions with the heel-palm. Make 30 circles then continue with the other side. This area is connected to the pericardium, where the 'chi reservoir' is to be found.

Benefits the heart, spleen and liver and circulation of chi to these organs.

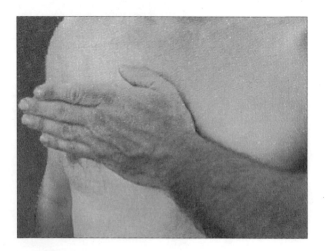

Head and face

In the exercises for the head we need to know
something of the pressure points. This first one is the
Baihui – which as we have seen is the middle point at
the top of the head. Apply pressure with the palm,
squeeze in with the fingers and then make gentle
circles. Repeat 40 times, 20 each way.

Benefits the brain and brain marrow, therefore
improving mental attributes such as clarity of thought
and memory.

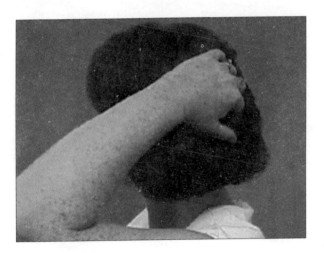

This next technique you will have used naturally for headaches.

Let the fingers rest against the forehead and the thumbs against the temples. Press moderately and make circular motions with the thumbs. These are the taiyang points through which, apart from headaches, we can influence facial pain and reduce blood pressure. Use approximately 30 circulations.

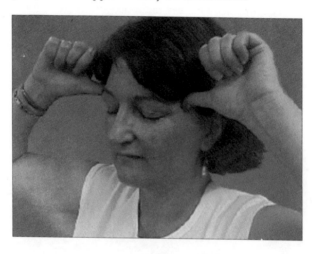

Chinese Medicine & Healthcare
Centre
24 Bernard Street, Leith
Edinburgh EH6 6PP
Tel. 0131 554 7888

For eyestrain and headaches related to eyestrain, use the following exercise.

Press with the index fingers on the points on the top of the nose, at the inner end of the eyebrows. Pull both hands outward, pressing on the eyebrows all the time. Repeat 20 times then do this next technique.

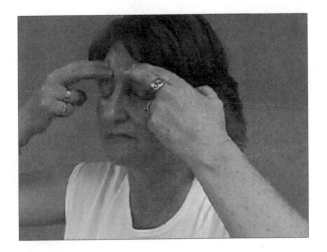

Starting at the same point as number 4 press down each side of the nose, repeating 20 times. This reduces facial pain, eases respiratory problems and helps clear the sinuses.

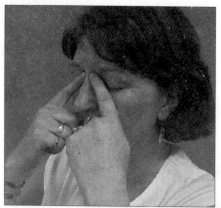

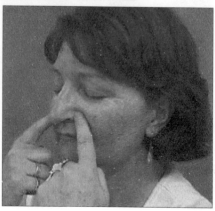

TUI means to push and is exactly what it implies. You can use thumb or palm, knuckle or elbow, but the technique must be smooth. Repeat the movement rhythmically using a constant pressure.

An ideal technique for those whose work involves repetitive physical activity, this technique removes toxic substances from the muscles and improves blood flow. Because of this it increases vitality and promotes balance.

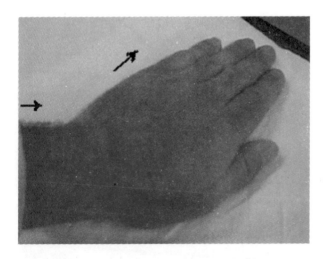

NA means grasping and twisting and can be used for most of the muscle groups. Use the thumb in opposition to the first two fingers or all if you prefer and create a pincer position. Grasp the body part in this way and twist to apply pressure, and then return to the original position (this action is like turning the key of a car). If the area requiring the action is an acupoint, squeeze then release. The wrist ought to be in a relaxed position throughout and the movements smooth and rhythmical.

This technique helps to release chi through the meridians creating a warming effect. It is excellent for relieving muscular pain and restoring regular function to the nervous system.

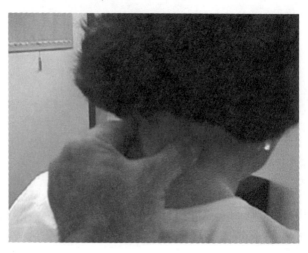

CHIA is a pinching technique and its primary use lies in the stimulation of acupoints. Using the thumb and index or thumb, index and middle fingers, apply strong pressure to the area requiring treatment, taking care not to cause damage to the tissues. Because it is a pinching action, this can be a painful technique, but do not use excessive pressure. Also useful in reducing swelling but again be sensible about the amount of pressure you use.

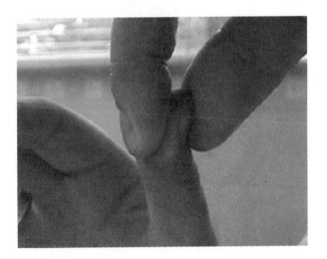

AN is simply pressure. Different areas require a different tool and with this technique we can use the palm, thumb, elbow, knuckle and fingers. Because of the action involved we need to practise this technique with a great deal of care. Using knuckle, thumb and/or finger pressure on an acupoint we can increase the pressure then hold for a few moments or use a rhythmic technique with half pressure. The same applies when we use the heel palm or elbow on the large muscle groups such as the upper back, chest, thighs and stomach.

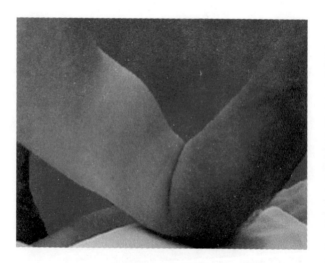

ROU is a technique much like kneading dough. We can use the same tools as we did for AN but instead of applying direct pressure we employ a circular motion, using a smooth but firm amount of force to the area requiring attention. Remember to keep the shoulders as relaxed as possible during the applications and the movements will remain even throughout.

Using palm or heel palm we can work on the area of the abdomen as an aid to the digestive tract, or use the elbow or double palm to reduce inflammation. As with AN the thumb, finger and knuckles can be used to adjust chi/blood flow.

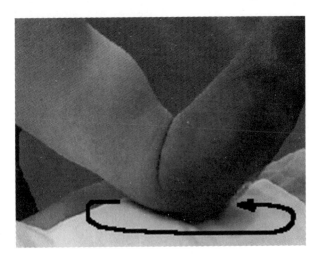

ZHEN is a powerful vibrating technique, which used on the muscles in order to reduce the affects of severe cramps. It can also be used to remove toxic substances from the blood after heavy workouts or hard physical labour.

Using the palms press deeply and vibrate along the muscle.

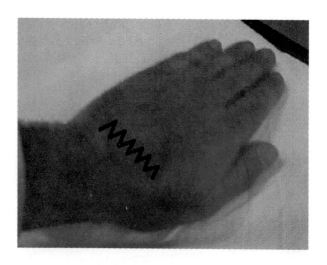

GUN is another technique for removing stress and toxic substances from the muscles. It has many of the benefits of ZHEN but its application is much gentler. Relax the hand as if holding a ball of cotton wool and roll over and back on the muscle. The more relaxed you are the more chi will pass through to the patient.

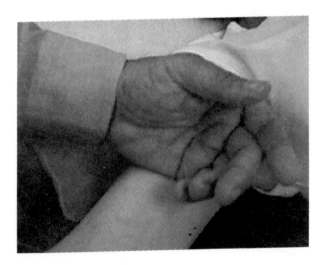

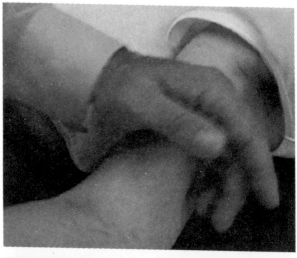

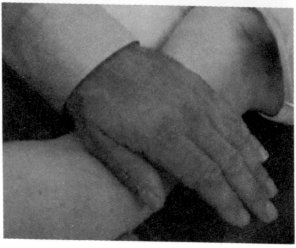

MOH is an extremely relaxing technique used to subdue and reduce excess energies. Using Thumbs and palms we press outwards, from the centre of the forehead to the temples, and then repeat until the patient feels calm. Apply to all areas of muscle trauma or where there is a blockage of chi.

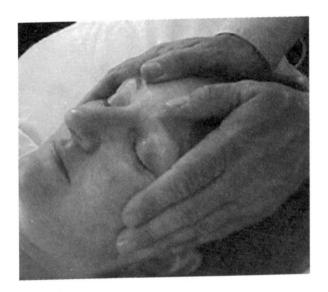

PAI and **KOU** are very similar techniques in that they use gentle striking actions to enhance the flow of chi/blood. PAI utilizes a tapping action with the front or back of the hand, or the fingers in a typing position. The movements are gentle and rhythmic and the technique can also be used on tender areas to relieve pain. KOU is a more robust action with the middle parts of the fingers of a lose fist. It employs a percussive, rhythmic action and is also excellent for removing tired energies.

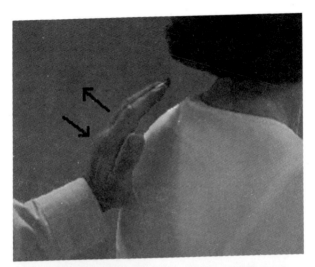

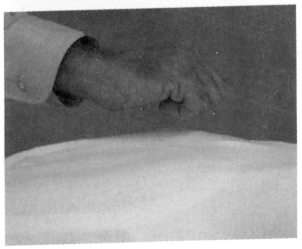

CUO is a twisting exercise for removing blockages to the free flow of chi/blood as well as toxic substances from the blood. Place the hands each side of the arm or leg and move one hand back while the other presses forward. Use a slight rolling action for the greatest benefit.

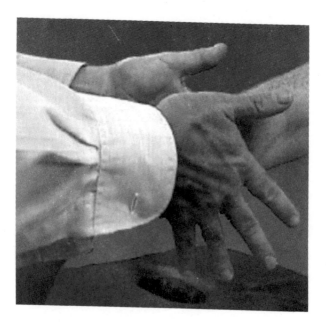

The next two techniques are primarily joint manipulations. **DOU** and **YAO** work together to remove tension and blocked energy from joints. DOU is a shaking action in which the arm or leg is shaken up and down like a towel. Hold the wrist and shoulder, tell the patient to relax, then shake gently from the wrist. This action also removes tired energies from the muscles. YAO is a simple turning action. Hold the wrist and forearm and utilize a circling action, or hold the wrist and above elbow or shoulder and use larger circles to work on the higher joints.

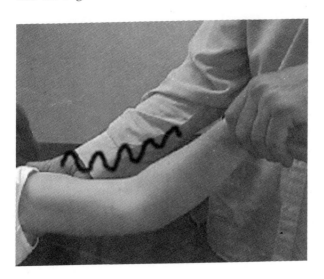

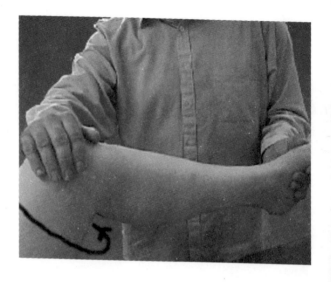

Much of tui-na manipulation is to relieve pain as well as treating the organs but its philosophy is the same as all of TCM, which is that 'prevention is preferable to cure'. It is suggested therefore that you engage the therapist in a regular whole-body session. Such a routine is outside the scope of this primer. If you interested in finding out more, we suggest you turn to the bibliography and purchase some of the examples you will find there.

Chapter five of Maria Mercati's Tui-na (see bibliog.) describes one such holistic treatment. Designed to prevent energy imbalances before disease can occur. The treatment restores balance on all levels, physical, mental and emotional, creating a sense of wholeness and well-being.

The book both demonstrates and teaches in a simple step-by-step manner, easy routines. The practical manner in which tui-na is presented makes it immediately accessible.

Peijian Shen's Massage for pain relief is equally practical, and includes an excellent chapter on simple self-massage, from which I have borrowed. Both of the above are highly recommended reading.

We can now move on to Chinese herbal therapies.

CHAPTER 8
TCM Herbalism

It is fundamental in a book of this type to plot the differences between Eastern and Western medicines, determining which is best according to the slant of the book. As we are attempting to accomplish a synthesis, it would be more profitable to observe the links between the two.

As laymen most of us might be forgiven if we believed, in an abstract way, that our Western pharmacology had little to do with plants and herbs. In fact many of us perceive our medicines to be entirely synthetic. While this is true to some extent, at least a quarter of our prescription drugs include extracts from herbs or plants.

Entering a chemist's shop, apart from toiletries etc, we are overwhelmed by brand name, colourfully produced, non-prescription treatments, most of which we will know. In the back of the shop we can usually observe shelves of prescription drugs, in anonymous boxes, whose use only the doctor and apothecary will know.

In a Chinese herbal remedy establishment we are greeted in an entirely different way. Jars containing plants, herbs, flowers and seeds line the shelves. Even the prepared formulas are recognisable as plant-based. Many of these we will know (in their English translation) from garden, field and hedgerow but again what we wont know is their use. If we were Chinese however, our TCM practitioner will probably have explained their use, how they were prepared and how and in what ways we will benefit.

Again, this is not to deprecate one form of medicine in favour of another. We can, however, begin to make the effort to find out a little more about this area of our own well-being. Many GP's now have a basic understanding (more in some cases) of holistic therapies. Take time where possible to discuss their replacement with modern drugs in your treatment. More importantly, discuss, read, and find out why.

There are other differences between modern drugs and herbal cures, especially TCM herbal remedies. One of the major differences occurs in their content. Most drugs tend to isolate the effective substance from the plant etc, while a TCM herbal treatment will use the whole plant, or group of plants. The purpose of which is to cushion the user against side effects, and/or increase the primary effect.

We cannot produce our own aspirin, but we can

begin to understand how to use nature for simple everyday remedies. There are alternatives to painkillers, diuretics, powerful drugs and inhalers. The use and composition of these alternatives might require a little work and cooperation from us: we may need to find someone with the knowledge, and be prepared to spend some time (and possibly money) to gain a basic understanding; we may even have to learn a little at a time what we are made up of, but this is the nature of independence. Without such a willingness to become responsible for our own well-being, there can be no self-sufficiency.

The sage-kings who compiled the I Ching and other classics, sought to master all areas of human endeavour. For them philosophy, psychology, self-protection (martial arts) and self-preservation (healing arts), were equal to and a part of, art and literature. It was the practical expression of human attributes, which dominated their philosophy.

The practitioner of TCM describes the complaint in simple terms to the patient: firstly in terms of yin and yang, excess and deficiency. The patient is then shown how to take part in his/her own recovery via simple self massage (acupressure techniques), and herbal treatments.

Next, the practitioner might expand his interpretation of the problem, to include five phase theory, explaining how the organ networks are affected. Finally he might broaden his prescription to incorporate diet and lifestyle: all of this so that firstly, the patient can take part in his/her own recovery, and secondly envision his/her life in holistic terms.

In Chinese Herbal Medicine an herb might be a plant, or it might be of mineral or animal material. It is prepared in such a way that the body can easily absorb and process it. Its purpose in traditional terms is to regulate the balance of blood, chi and fluids via the organ networks. It will do so by expelling the five outside evils (cold, wind, heat, damp and dryness/summer heat) and balancing the five emotions (anger, joy, pensiveness, fear/fright and sadness/grief).

A Chinese herbalist tailors the prescription to suit the individual, according to his/her diagnosis. This prescription could include few or many different herbs. Each of these herbs is chosen for one or more of its various qualities. There are literally thousands of herbs in use, each of which exhibits one or more effective uses – effective in the manner of re-establishing harmony. It is not surprising therefore that prescriptions vary.

It is not the function of this book to provide recipes or cures from what is a complex tradition. If anything we have attempted to create a simple overview of the subject. We think it would be more helpful, in this respect, to illustrate the vast array of herbs via their qualitative uses.

The two primary categories for herbs in TCM refer

to their temperature and taste.

The five temperature characteristics are:

- Cold, hot, warm, cool and neutral.

The five taste characteristics are:

- Sweet, spicy, sour, bitter and salt.

Taste and temperature combine to create the properties by which the herbs effectively re-establish balance within the body. The temperature of the herb describes its action on the individual and his/her condition. This means, for instance, that a warming herb will be used to treat cold conditions; a cooling herb will be used for excess heat and so on.

The taste of the herb directs the healing action to the corresponding organ network. (The five tastes connect with the five phases and therefore the five organ networks.)

Sour links with wood, and 'heals' the liver and the gall-bladder.
Bitter links to fire, the heart and small intestine.
Sweet to earth, stomach and spleen.
Spicy to metal, lungs and large intestine.
Salt to water, kidney and bladder.

Herbs can also combine and break-up, purge and tonify.
These categories imply the following effects:
When an herb has a combining quality it is able to

concentrate the chi, blood and fluids, inhibiting the leakage of bodily materials through discharge, excess tears, sweating, urination etc.

To break-up implies the opposite: that where there is stagnation of chi, blood and fluids, the density will be broken up. This frees the circulatory processes and disperses the harmful build up.

To purge means simply to eject. When the herb has broken-down the harmful blockage, it will then expel the harmful substances. An herb of this type will be used for blockages such as cysts and tumours.

An herb used for tonifying is able to reinforce the body, after other herbs have broken down blockages and driven out the toxic substances. Primarily they generate chi, blood and fluids to enhance the body's resistance after illness etc.

Some herbal formulas and their general applications

It should be noted that most professionals use a basic formula, which they will then customise for the individual patient. For those engaged in regular hard training, visiting a TCM practitioner with a view to receiving a concoction, based on personal constitution and climate, is the best course. For some of the more common ailments we might want to have an herb store at home.

When dealing with symptoms of cold and flu, use the medication in early stages for best benefits.

The following formulas and teas are designed for general use only and can be purchased at most Chinese Herbal Establishments. Always ask for the advice from the herbalist, and follow the instructions with care.

Zheng gu shui
In liniment form – good for bruising and minor fractures. Reduces pain from general sports injuries.

Xiao huo luo dan
In pill form, used mainly for strains and bone damage. Can also be used for general aches and pains.

Bai hua yu
In oil form, this is primarily for stiffened muscles and strains. Can irritate the eyes so apply carefully.

Tian chi jiu
A liniment used mainly for bruises and contusions.

Yunnan bai yao
In powder form, this concoction stops bleeding immediately. It also promotes healing little scarring. Used mainly for minor cuts and scrapes.

Yu ping feng san
One of many concoctions for hay-fever, this is recommended as a combined treatment with acupuncture for swift relief. The acupuncture is used firstly to remove the blockages and restore balance. This is followed by the herbal remedy to aid in strengthening the wei chi (protective chi).

Yin Chao Chieh Tu Pien
An ancient remedy used primarily for the common cold. It is said to expel heat and wind, which cause the problem. To be used in the early stages of the attack. Can also be used to combat allergies.

Lo Han Kuo
For symptoms including dry coughs and thirst, this delicious concoction alleviates the sore throat by

diminishing the dryness.

Ching Chi Hua Tan Wan
When the cough produces phlegm this formula is
more suitable.

Wu Chai Pai Feng
Mainly used by women to ease menstruation
difficulties, such as cramps, exhaustion, mood
changes and irregularity.

Chieh Keng T'ang
This expectorant is mostly for problems of the throat
such as tonsillitis and laryngitis.

Chih Kan Ts'ao T'ang
Stimulates and strengthens the heartbeat when the
pace is weak, irregular or racing.

Ch'ing Chieh Lien Chih T'ang
This formula stimulates and strengthens the liver.
Good for acne, baldness and mental difficulties.

Hsiao Chien Chung T'ang
A tonic to relieve exhaustion. Also for bedwetting.

Kan Ts'ao Fu Tzu T'ang
A diuretic for the treatment of joint problems such as
arthritis and rheumatism.

Ke Ken T'ang
A most excellent concoction for the internal organs, this one strengthens, kidneys, liver, heart and intestines.

Li Mo T'ang
For the treatment of stomach and throat problems.

Pai Hu Chia Jen Shen T'ang
Also known as 'white tiger tea' this is an outstanding brew for generating harmony.

Su Tzu Chiang Ch'i T'ang
A diuretic for treating kidney problems, caused by an excess of yang, such as ulcers and rashes.

Wi Chi San
Another all-rounder – for chi and water diseases; treats anemia and stomach problems, as well as menstrual pain and pelvic difficulties.

Yin Ch'en Wu Ling San
A diuretic; treats internal organs such as gall bladder, liver and kidneys. Good for gallstones, jaundice and constipation.

Also for problems such as:

allergies	**Bi Yan Pian**
asthma	**Ma Hsing Yi Kan T'ang**
blood pressure (high)	**Fang Feng T'ung Sheng San**
blood pressure (low)	**Pu Chung Yi Ch'i T'ang**
constipation	**Mu Xiang Shen Chi Wan**
diabetes	**Ta Ch'ai Hu T'ang**
diarrhoea	**Liu Jun Zi Wan** has fast results
dysentery	**Ta Huang Mu T'ang**
eczema	**Kuei Chih Fu Ling Wan**
epilepsy	**Ch'ai Hu Chia Lung Ku Mu Li T'ang**
food poisoning	**Yin Ch'en Kao T'ang**
hernia	**Ch'ai Hu Kuei Chih T'ang**
impotence	**Pa Wei Wan**
mastitis	**Ke Ken T'ang**
migraine	**Yan Hu Suo** is good
muscular spasms	**Hsiao Yao Wan** also has good effects
myopia	**Ling Kuei Shu Kan T'ang**
piles	**Yi Tzu Tang /Pu Chung Yi Ch'I T'ang**
pneumonia	**Hsao Ch'ai Hu T'ang**
rheumatics	**Chi Ye Lien**
sore throats	**Pan Hsia Hsieh Hsin T'ang**
uterine cysts	**Ts'ao Ho Ch'eng Ch'I T'ang**
worms	**Ke Ken T'ang**

How to prepare a herbal tea or formula

There are many ways of preparing Chinese herbal teas but the following is one of the preferred methods.

Use a glass or ceramic container with a lid. Do not use metal, plastic or aluminium pots as these can interact with the herbs. At best this will spoil the tea and at worst have a negative effect on the drinker.

A formula will consist of between a half and two ounces of materials and three to six cups of water. Leave to soak for a quarter-hour then cook them from twenty minutes to an hour. When there is about a cupful left pour out the liquid and repeat, using the same herbs.

Mix the contents of both steepings together. This is because in the first steeping the temperature energetic is drawn from the herb, while the second time it is the taste energetic. The former affects the chi, the latter the blood.

There is a difference in cooking time due to the ease or difficulty in extracting the ingredients required. Where oils are concerned, these will evaporate quickly once extracted, so a short time is required. It could also be that some herbs in the formula require longer than others. If this is so we can cook separately.

It may not always be necessary to cook the herbs, sometimes just adding boiling water is sufficient to remove the therapeutic ingredients.

Once cooked we must now employ correct timing

for their ingestion. Obviously if you have received the formula from a TCM practitioner, she/he will have included this information with the ingredients. If not then, generally, the following is suggested:

If there is no reason to the contrary, an hour before meals on an empty stomach.

If problems such as mild stomach upset occur, drink an hour after meals, or use a little fresh ginger or ginger juice before drinking.

CHAPTER 9

T'ai Chi Chuan and Chi Gung

T'ai Chi Chuan is currently performed primarily for its martial and health aspects, though it is achieving respect for its purely callisthenics qualities. It is known as an internal martial art, because of its emphasis on the development of Chi as opposed to muscular training.

As with Chi Gung, with which there is a direct connection, the movements concentrate energy on the organs and systems of the body. The Chi is encouraged to flow more readily through the channels, (or meridians) to ensure a balanced system.

In the practise of T'ai Chi Chuan, the first emphasis is on the external forms. There are many reasons for this: for instance the free flow of internal energy depends on physical co-ordination. More importantly however, is the part that the conscious mind must play: the mind must control the movements from the centre. This centre is located just below the navel, and so awareness must be there.

This exercise requires constant practise before proficiency is achieved, but once it is, all of our activities begin to take on a new and harmonious significance.

The centre and consciousness must attempt to become one: to move in unison but the lower centre guided by the upper centre. This principle originates in the I Ching: the second and fifth lines symbolise centres in the upper and lower trigrams: for there to be natural balance, the higher self must direct the lower self, but only from a position of unity.

The lower centre is Yin and therefore relates to the earth: we encourage this by sinking. This is done by relaxing the muscles and allowing the joints to move freely: this in turn allows more energy to circulate through the various channels: blood, breath and Chi sink toward the earth, providing relaxed power at the centre. The principle we call sinking might also be termed grounding, in that, we are consciously aligning ourselves with the force of gravity. Strange as this might sound, once we have become accustomed to this we find we are far more relaxed mentally and emotionally. This is because we are no longer pressing ourselves away from the ground.

The body is aligned in a particular way: the head supported by the spine, the spine by the pelvic girdle, then through the legs to the feet, which support all.

In T'ai Chi, learning to carry the body this way with the joints relaxed and open, breath sunk into the centre, creates an excellent sense of well being.

Once the consciousness enters into the centre and we achieve this sense of harmony, we begin to recognise the difference between responding and reacting.

When the lower centre moves without the control of the upper centre i.e. the conscious mind, this is called a reaction. An objective mind responds calmly and clearly to a given situation: the speed of response depends entirely on the situation (see Chian Long Classic below).

When the lower centre moves in a reactionary way, it is the instincts that are directing it. This is explained in the I Ching in the following way: the third line, symbolising our desires, emotional reactions or instincts, presses down and seeks to control the lower functions, (symbolised by the two lower lines) by blocking energy from the fifth line. The imbalance created by this causes disease and lack of harmony in the whole structure- creating fear, the need for more control, and so on.

With practise we begin to understand that the energy of Chi (Prana, Ki or Lifeforce) is as immediate as our thoughts. When the conscious mind and the body are correctly attuned (i.e. to the present moment), all of our activities are filled with a vitality and resonance we have not experienced since early childhood.

Practising forms at such a slow pace requires great

discipline of mind to begin with: learning the principles of movement, balance and relaxation, as well as co-ordinating emptiness and fullness can be extremely demanding. Each time the form is practised the mind is continuously alert for areas requiring improvement: this also includes negative reactions such as impatience and boredom.

After the forms have been mastered, the internal energy begins to pass through the body and limbs as a result of the conscious will. As the physical co-ordination improves, channelling the energy from the heels through the waist to the upper limbs becomes effortless.

It is important, in T'ai Chi training, to learn the method (forms) as well as the principles, but if we focus on one at the expense of the other, our practise will be meaningless.

In Chen style T'ai Chi this imperative is no more important than in learning the Chan Si Gung, or Silk Reeling method. This method of movement, and the inner force produced during the practise of it, can only be mastered when we can adequately apply the principle of sinking to all the joints, and consciously direct all movements from the centre.

In T'ai Chi terms, employing Yin means to make oneself empty, whereas Yang means making oneself full: Yin is gentleness, Yang is forcefulness.

T'ai Chi Chuan Classic of the Chian-Long Dynasty (1736–1796)

Chang San Feng is one of those credited with creation of T'ai Chi Chuan, and it was he who wrote the original treatise in the Song dynasty (960–1127 AD). Many masters of the art have formulated their own account of this text and the above named classic is one of them.

In translating ancient T'ai Chi texts we are met with two difficulties. Firstly the scope of its philosophy is so vast: at one extreme T'ai Chi, viewed in its simple form is a slow dance; while in its more complex and esoteric extreme it is representative of the evolution of the Cosmos. (On the one hand structure, on the other meaning.)

The second difficulty is simpler and arises out of changes in writing style in the past 200 years. As with all languages, alterations in Chinese have occurred as a result of the advancement of culture, and so it is with no surprise that we can observe vast differences in the numerous translations.

In the Ye family tradition the practise of T'ai Chi is really quite simple: play it like a slow dance. The more you train, the more you will want to train, and the more you will understand how and why you train.

The theory in the Classic of the Chian Long Dynasty appears to be in the form of a map, which prepares the newcomer by offering simple guidance. If you have the map there is no need to remember as a result of study, simply use it to check your movements each time you train. You will assimilate it with practise.

The following is the translation with amendments, by Professor Zude Ye, of the T'ai Chi Classic of the Chian Long Dynasty. I offer this to show the reader the simple view, concerning the movement of Chi, in the original texts.

> For the Chi to move along the neck to the crown of the head it is essential to relax the shoulders.
> The Chi then sinks to the Tan Tien (lower abdomen) and is guided along the thighs and hips.
> The Ha sound emitted from the Tan Tien extends the Jing (energy), strengthening the fists.
> The five toes grasp the ground the back (top of the body) is bent like a bow.

(The following teaches about still standing posture.)

> Inhale to Tan Tien.
> Transfer Chi to sacrum then up to crown via the neck.
> Then down front of body to thighs, lower legs and toes.

The Zhong or still standing posture of T'ai Chi is the basic for a firm stance and the free flow of the Chi.

During motion be light and agile and condense the spirit hidden within (the whole body).

Move continuously so that the Chi flows steadily.

When the intention is to move to the right, the first movement is to the left and vice versa.

If the movement is up then the intention is to first go down. Again the reverse applies.

To refine the internal Gung Fu the key is in the Tan Tien.

Hin and Ha the two Chi's are infinite.

Chi separates to yin and yang in movement and unites in stillness.

Follow your opponent, if he extends you bend- or the reverse. Slow responds to slow, fast to fast.

These principles must be thoroughly understood.

Suddenly appear or disappear, moving forward but no more than an inch.

Regarding balance, even one feather added may break it and the Tao is hidden within it.

Hands move slow or fast depending on the situation.

When this principle is practised and understood four ounces can deflect a thousand pounds.

(The next two parts are strategies for combat.)
Be prepared for changes.
Whether forward back left or right do not move to excess. The key is balance.
Speed depends on the opponent. Borrow his force to defeat him.
Hen sound comes from the lungs and links with the nose. Ha sound comes from the stomach and links with the mouth.

Wardoff rollback press and push are the primary directions.
Pluck split elbow and shoulder are the four corners.
There are eight kua or trigrams corresponding to the I Ching which are kan, k'un, chen, sun, chien, tui, ken, and li.
Forward, back left, right, rear and centre represent the five elements.

Extremely soft means hardness. Like a needle hidden within cotton.
Move as if drawing silk but be clear about your direction.
Open and extending, tight and compact one

upon the other; movements should be threaded together tightly.

When there is an opportunity for action move like the cat.

(And so the strategies for action are:)

Hard is to be found in softness like a needle hidden in cotton.

Movement is like drawing silk.

Action mimics the cat.

Change begins with a careful mind.

Translated by Professor Zude Ye

Chinese Medicine & Healthcare
Centre
24 Bernard Street, Leith
Edinburgh EH6 6PP
Tel. 0131 554 7888

Chi Gung

Chi Gung is an ancient Chinese art and science, by which the practitioner develops and cultivates the life force (Chi) by effort and practise (Gung). Exercises are performed through sequential movements like those of T'ai Chi (soft Chi Gung), or Gung Fu forms (hard Chi Gung). They can be practised as single techniques, sitting or standing, lying down or as sexual alchemy.

Chi Gung can be performed quietly as in meditation, or with the use of sound, as in a technique known as six healing sounds.

There are such a huge variety of systems, each with its own arsenal of techniques, that it would be impractical to attempt a comprehensive study of Chi Gung. Of primary importance, for the interested student, is finding a good teacher. This is not as difficult as it used to be, though it is worth spending some time in research, both of the material and the teacher. Invest in one or two books on the subject.

The original system was called Nei Gung, which means internal development through effort. These were predominantly meditational exercises, used by Taoist sage-kings (see chapter on I Ching), whose primary purpose was to increase spiritual understanding and power. The fact that these exercises also maintained and regained superior health, and improved fighting abilities, was secondary.

Some useful Chi Gung exercises

The following Chi Gung exercises are practised for a variety of purposes, all of which, as you would expect, relate to health. In all of the following and indeed in all Chi Gung exercises, there are three primary ingredients, which are movement, breath and intention. Firstly we learn to move, then to move with breath, and finally to move with breath and intention.

Once this has been achieved, a Chi Gung exponent no longer needs the movements: he/she can circulate the energy in time with the breath. Mastery is when the Chi can be moved by concentration alone. Simply by imagining the chi flowing from the tantien to the fingers results in an immediate flush of energy.

In practising (and practise means only, to actively repeat) Chi gung exercises we are breaking down destructive blockages, by freeing productive energy processes.

Still standing stance

This first exercise both balances and awakens the Chi, while calming those other energies. This is the still standing stance, which is also known as, standing like a child. (Shan Shuang).

Stand with the feet about shoulder width apart, the weight is evenly distributed. Relax the knees and hips slightly so that the joints are open. It is not necessary to sink to a position where the stance becomes painful or uncomfortable.

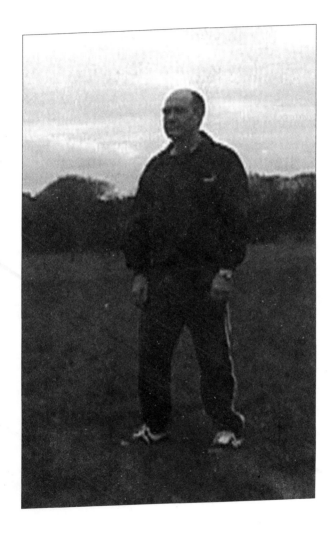

Raise the elbows until they are in line with the ribs, and turned down as if they were too heavy to lift. The forearms extend to the front with the hands turned slightly inward, wrists relaxed. Again the joints are thrown open. This is to aid the free flow of Chi, throughout the body.

The head is erect without the neck being stiff. Imagine that there is a cord from the ceiling to the crown of the head. This gives the body a feeling of being light and suspended.

The spine is straight, but relaxed. The shoulders are also relaxed, which allows the chest to sink. This in turn allows the centre of gravity to sink to the abdomen. Breathe gently from the lower stomach, the place known as the TanTien.

Finally close the eyes and allow the tongue to touch the roof of the mouth.

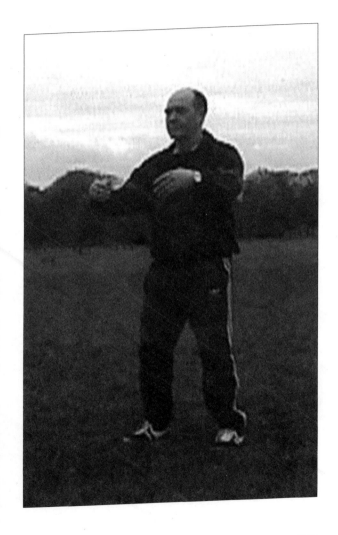

Standing this way for about fifteen minutes enables the unbalanced energies to sink to the TanTien, where they become balanced. If practised regularly, you will sense your inner tensions immediately, and release them.

This is an excellent way to start the day, especially if your day is likely to be stressful.

The time can slowly be extended up to about half an hour, after which you can add any or all of the following exercises if you wish.

When standing still try to imagine the energy of the earth (gravity if you like) entering the body through the meridians of the feet. When you feel that you can visualize this, imagine also that the energy of the cosmos enters through the crown of the head and the palms of the hands. This is not meant to be a wilful exercise but one in which you feel yourself to be a part of the world and the universe.

The end product of all chi gung and t'ai chi exercises is that we learn to 'let go' of the destructive patterns of thought and behaviour. Remember the breath – remember to relax.

When speaking of Chi gung, the ancient Daoists would say, 'Standing still, doing nothing'. Master Chen Xiaowang says, 'Stand like a mountain. This is most important'.

The first exercise balances disturbed energies,

whereas this next one awakens the Chi, allowing it to flow freely through the channels.

Opening Stance

Stand as in the Shan Shuang stance, feet shoulder
width apart, but with both arms hanging at your side.

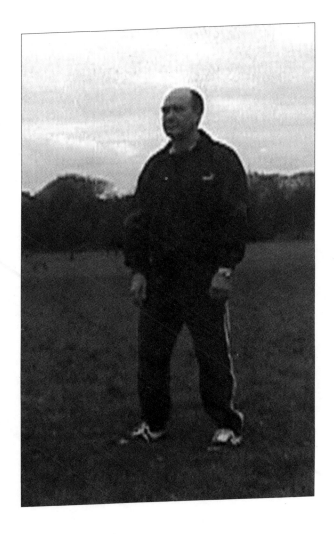

Relax shoulders and hips, then, allow both arms to float to shoulder level.

The elbows point down and the wrists are relaxed. As the hands reach shoulder level, extend the hands and the Chi will rise to the fingers.

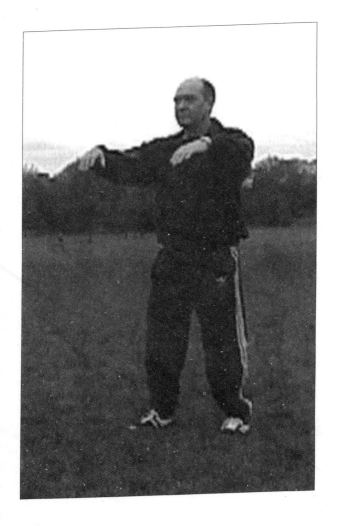

Next let the shoulders relax, so that the elbows fall to the sides.

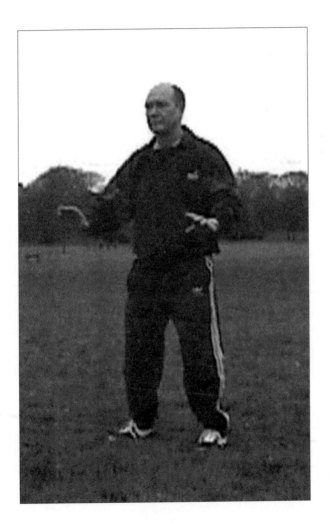

Now the elbows relax and finally the fingers. The hands are now at the sides again.

Repeat the exercise twenty times. Hold the position for half a minute, between each repetition, to allow the Chi to settle in the TanTien.

During the exercise imagine that you are in a swimming pool. Let the arms float up to shoulder level, breathing lightly into the TanTien, and as they float down, breathe out.

After a period of practise the fingers will tingle and the hands begin to get warm. These are manifestations (effects) of chi.

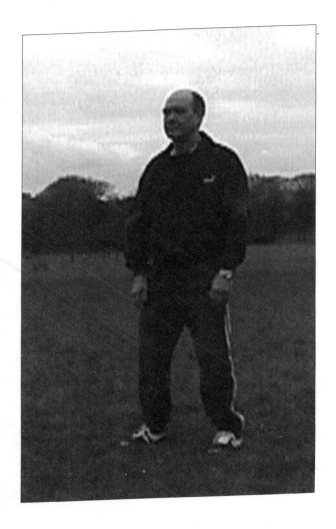

Grounding exercise

The final exercise of this group can be used as a grounding exercise. It is a simple way of closing the doors after a session of Chi Gung. This is the exercise I use after a T'ai Chi session.

Use the shoulder width stance, with the arms hanging loosely at the sides.

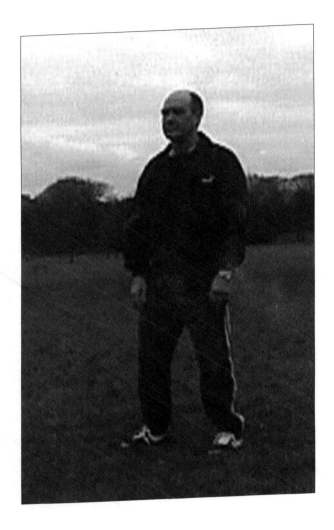

As you breathe in, let the arms lift gently stretched out to the sides until they reach shoulder height, palms down.

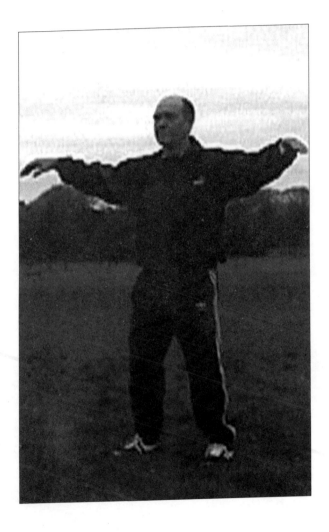

Continuing to breathe in, turn the palms over...

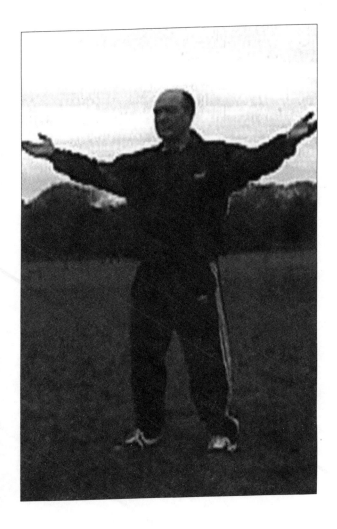

...and bring them almost together above your head.

This part of the movement is performed a little faster. As before the breathing is into the Tantien, or the lower abdomen.

The elbows bend outwards, allowing the hands to sink to head height, then slowly down past the face and chest to the sides again. The breathe from above the head is out. Repeat the exercise for about twenty repetitions with ten seconds pause between each.

During the out breath of the above exercise, as the hands pass the face tell the muscles to relax. The same with the throat, chest, and solar plexus. Finally relax the abdomen, then the legs, all the way to the ground as the hands turn to the sides again.

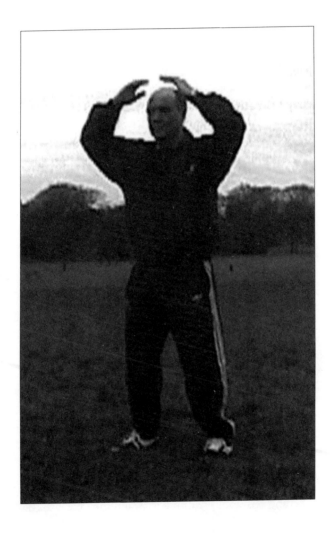

With every repetition do the same with other parts of the body: so when we are at head height again, begin with the scalp, back of the neck, shoulders etc, relaxing the back as the hands fall past the chest and abdomen.

Once this is done, and you feel as if all the body is in a relaxed state, imagine closing the entrances to the main acupuncture points, beginning of course with the Baihui. The hands are in the position above the head and we are about to breathe out. As we allow the breath to leave and the hands sink to within an inch of the scalp, we concentrate on closing the door to the energy centre. Hold for about ten seconds before moving to the next point.

(The purpose of this part of the exercise is, as I have said, to close the doors. This is to prevent leakage of energy from these areas.)

Close the doors by telling them to close. (In Chi Gung we are gaining conscious control of our energy input and output.)

After the Bai hui point, move to the Yintang, the point between the eyebrows. Concentrate, and then move to Ren22, (the hollow just above the breastbone) Ren 17 (centre of breastbone between the nipples) and Ren 14, (six inches above the navel) in the same way; finally Ren 4 (three inches below the navel). It will not be possible to close all of these points in one movement, we will have to return to the opening position, breathing in again, then back to the

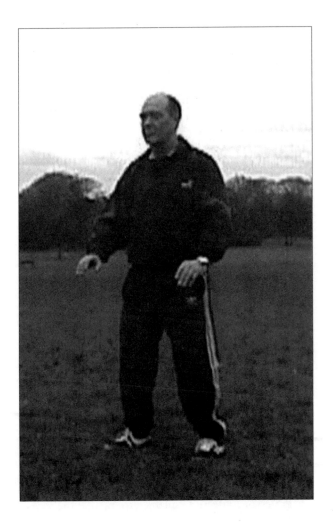

head and down. If you feel comfortable closing one at a time, then repeating the whole exercise to reach the next position, this works equally well.

Finally begin to close the back positions. Raising the hands to the head let them fall behind to the occipital ridge to Du16 (the hollow under the occipital ridge); then to the spine at a point between the shoulder blades Du14. This last is a little uncomfortable at first but persevere with it.

Allowing the hands to fall to the sides, lift them behind the back to a place parallel, and a little lower, to the navel, the Mingmen orDu4. The final point is Du1, midpoint between the anus and genitals. This is the acupuncture point called Hui Yin, and it is necessary to close this gate after practising Chi Gung. The closing exercise is simple and involves a contraction of the anus and genitals. This contraction is repeated three times, while concentrating on the closure.

The exercise in itself is finished and it remains only to relax for about a minute, while the Chi sinks to the TanTien.

As you can imagine, something formulated over thousands of years, cannot be learned in a day. This is true about Chi Gung; but it is only the knowledge involved in this discipline, which cannot be learned quickly.

Professor Zude Yee explained to me that the

exercises we call Chi Gung, are observations of natural phenomena, made by generations of healers. These observations went through stringent tests, to prove their authenticity, before being passed on scrupulously.

Do not sit down immediately after Chi Gung exercises, stand in the still standing stance, this time with the hands at the sides, or walk around and perform light tasks. Do this for about five minutes, by which time the Chi will have settled.

Chi gung is a primary component of TCM and we recommend that the interested reader find a competent instructor. An excellent introductory book (among many), is Sandra Hill's, Reclaiming the Body. There are exercises for each of the internal organs, and the interpretation of five phase theory and practise is simple and easy to follow.

CHAPTER 10
A Brief Summary of TCM

The subject of Traditional Chinese Medicine could of course fill volumes: each of its individual components is a lengthy study in itself.

As with the other Eastern traditions, TCM is a holistic therapy. As we have seen, amongst its vast array of health care practices is breath and movement techniques; herbal, diet and massage therapies; acupuncture, acupressure and healing sound treatments. The list is exhaustive.

TCM is fundamentally Shamanism, and its principles are based on the philosophy of the I Ching. The interaction between the forces of heaven and earth, and man's ability to consciously use these forces, provide the basis for a system of self-development and health.

The energies are called yin (for earth), and yang (for heaven), and disease is seen as an imbalance between these two.

Yin is perceived as the denser of the two energies,

and links us to the world. Yin energy is expressed through food and drink, rest and the accumulation of energy. In a healthy way, Yin allows us calm detachment from objects, in order that Yang the primordial energy, can find expression in the world.

When Yin has become imbalanced, it is because we have become attached to the world, in a manner that blocks out the free passage of Yang energy.

Yang, in everyday terms, is healthily expressed through ordinary activities, which benefit our society as a whole: the simple happiness we experience in helping others is an expression of Yang in the world.

Yang becomes unhealthy when we are conscious of our actions and fall into the trap of observing self. In this condition we fall prey to habitual thought patterns and the demands that accompany them.

These demands manifest in many ways: overindulgence in food and drink, which quite often develops into the opposite as we become aware of the effects and move from one extreme to the other, in an effort to control the excess.

We overspend or hoard money in the search for satisfaction; feed our vanities with ever-increasing demands on others and ourselves. The list is endless and encompasses the greatest proportion of human misery.

Health in TCM means fundamentally:

To be well, we need to be whole: to be whole means to know what we are made up of.

Sun Tsu in the Art of War tells us that success depends on,

'Knowing the enemy and knowing oneself':

Sometimes our most dangerous enemy is within self.

The I Ching separates the human mind and the mind of Tao, or Universal mind. This does not mean that they describe two disparate entities, only that they are dissimilar levels of the conscious mind, each having its own activity. Problems occur when one seeks to subjugate the other.

TCM is a practical system of health, a holistic system with a simple base: well-being occurs when Yin is Yin, and Yang is Yang. The primary purpose of TCM is prevention of disease, and only in a secondary sense is it viewed as a cure.

When the human mind (Yin) controls the Universal mind (Yang) imbalance (disease) is expressed in our whole being. And equally, when Yang seeks to control the lower functions, misery occurs.

It is the interaction, between the primary forces of

Yin and Yang that results in change. Change is the path of development: comprehending and plotting this path leads to health.

In the evolutionary process of I Ching and TCM philosophy, the Chinese sages observed how the primary forces operated in the seasons.

In spring Yang was present as vital energy, an awakening life force, overcoming the death-grip of winter. In summer, as Yang reached its zenith, in a flourish of energy, they detected the faintest movement of Yin. Autumn was the unfolding of Yin, and the withdrawing of Yang. Finally, as the cold of winter prevailed over the world, Yin was in the ascendant.

Spring was dubbed young Yang; summer old Yang; autumn was young Yin and winter old yin.

This was how the interaction of forces manifested to create change in the world.

Spring signified the first outward movement, an expansion, while summer was an extension of energy, upward. In autumn there was a contraction, while winter entailed a downward, resting movement. These movements occurred about the world and so each was assigned a direction.

- Spring outward to the east.
- Summer up and to the south.
- Autumn a sinking of energy and to the west.
- Winter a downward movement to the north.
  With earth at the centre, these became the five

stages (movements) of change. (Often incorrectly called elements of change).

From these five stages, and their attributes, was generated an intricate methodology for combating disease.

The five phases were symbolised by earth, wood, fire, metal and water. The characteristics of the five symbols of change were then assigned to the five major organs, and the emotions that spring from them.

The organs produce, change and control the Chi (Ki, Universal energy), as well as the blood, via channels throughout the body. As regards the Chi, these channels are called meridians.

The sage healers concluded also that the spiritual aspect of the individual manifested through the organs, in a variety of ways. The word for spirit in Chinese is shen, which can be singular or plural. Singularly it is the spirit governing the heart, whereas in a collective sense it represents the spiritual aspects of all of the organs.

This can seem quite confusing, but if we take it to signify spiritual qualities, rather than entities, we can apprehend the meaning more easily.

Taoist healers observed that when the quality of spirit was strong, the body, thought patterns and emotions were both healthy and strong.

In conclusion, I will repeat that the primary purpose of TCM is to achieve balance of the primal energies, preferably before the onset of disease. This is the simplicity of its methodology, evident in herbal medicine, Tai Chi, acupuncture, diet and chi gung.

A Simple Chronology

FuHsi 2852 BC
The origin of TCM and formulation of yin/yang
theory. Also credited with formulating I Ching (book
of changes).

Shen Nung c2697 BC
Shen Nung'S Herbal.

Huang Ti 2697–2595 BC
Inventor – currency, ships, musical notation. Wrote
the Huang Ti Nei Ching. (The Yellow Emporer's
Classic of Internal Medicine).

240 AD or earlier
The Tso Chuan, a stone-carved historical record
contains many medical references.

Tsou Yen c305–240 BC
Attempted combination of Ayurvedic (Indian) with

TCM. Developed Wu Hsing or five phase theory.

Chang Chung Ching (the Chinese Hippocrates) c158–166 AD

Created system of yin/yang symptom characteristics. Wrote Shang Han Lun (Treatise on ailments caused by cold).

Hua To c136–141 AD

A surgeon and acupuncturist, he studied anatomy and physical therapy. He introduced antiseptics and anaesthesia. He developed methods of physical activity known as the five animals, which eventually evolved into the Chinese martial arts as we know them today.

Ko Hung 281–340 AD

Wrote Chin Kuei Yo Fang (Medications from the Golden Box) and Chou-Hou Pei-Tsi Fang (First Aid). Included a chapter on cheap, easy to find medical recipes.

T'ao Hung Ching 452–536 AD

Wrote and edited an annotated Shen Nung Pen Ts'ao.

Sun Szu Miao 582–682 AD

His major work was the 1000 recipes or Ts'ien Chin Fang to which he also wrote a supplement.

Li Shih Chen 1518–1593

The Pen Ts'ao Kang Mu, an extensive volume of
material medica ranking with the Nei Ching and
Shang Han.

Bibliography

Massage for Pain Relief, Peijian Shen. Gaia Books, London 1996.

Step by Step Tuina, Maria Mercati. Gaia Books, London 1997.

Reclaiming the Wisdom of the Body, Sandra Hill. Constable and Co., London 1997.

Between Heaven and Earth (A guide to Chinese medicine), Harriet Beinfield L.Ac. and Efrem Korngold L.Ac., O.M.D.. Ballantine books, New York 1991.

Chinese Medicine, Tom Williams Ph.D. Element Books, Dorset 1995.

Chinese Herbal Medicine (Ancient art and modern science), Richard Hyatt with Therapeutic Repertory by Robert Feldman M.D. Wildwood Hse. Ltd., London 1978.

Acupuncture (The modern scientific approach), Anthony Campbell MRCP (UK), FF Hom. Faber and Faber, London 1987.

Acupuncture (Cure of many diseases), Felix Mann, MB, Bchir (Cambridge). Butterworth Heinemann Ltd., Oxford, 1971.

Alternative Therapies, Edited by G.T. Lewith, MA, MRCP, MRCGP. William Heinemann Medical BOOKS Ltd. London 1985.

Complementary Medicine Today (Practitioners and Patients), Ursula Sharma. Routledge, London 1992.

I Ching or Book of Changes, Richard Wilhelm translation, rendered into English by Cary F. Baynes. Routledge and Kegan Paul Ltd, London 1951.

The Alternative Health Guide, Brian Inglis and Ruth West. Michael Joseph, London 1983.

Complementary and Alternative Medicine, Marc S. Micozzi with a foreword by C. Everett Koop. Churchill Livingstone 1996.

Also the following from www.
Al Stone L.Ac Santa Monica West Hollywood CA